Trauma Centers

Jeffrey S. Young

Trauma Centers

A Quick Guide

Foreword by J. Wayne Meredith

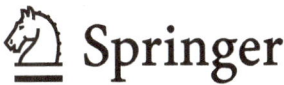 Springer

Jeffrey S. Young
Troy, VA
USA

ISBN 978-3-030-34606-5   ISBN 978-3-030-34607-2   (eBook)
https://doi.org/10.1007/978-3-030-34607-2

This Springer imprint is published by the registered company Springer Nature Switzerland AG
The registered company address is: Gewerbestrasse 11, 6330 Cham, Switzerland

This work is dedicated to all the prehospital, emergency department, operating room, intensive care unit, acute care, and rehabilitation personnel who care for the injured patient.

Foreword

I have known Jeff Young since he started his internship at Wake Forest University in 1988. Since that time, I have been happy to be his mentor and friend. He followed many of the steps I took in my career including becoming a trauma director at a university hospital; becoming involved in the American College of Surgeons Committee on Trauma, becoming an experienced and busy site review for the verification review committee; and progressing through leadership roles in national trauma organizations.

Even though there are many trauma centers and many people who work in them, no one has taken the time to write out the basic principles and processes to progress from a hospital to a trauma center. Dr. Young has done this admirably, and this handbook will be of use to administrators, surgeons, fellows, nurses, and anyone deeply involved in trauma center care. Dr. Young's extensive experience performing site visits for the ACS allows him a unique perspective that all centers will find helpful.

I hope that you will take the time to read this handbook and recommend it to all who may benefit from it. Saving the injured is a calling, and doing it better every day is a profession. This handbook will help you do both.

J. Wayne Meredith, MD
Richard T. Myers Professor and Chair
Department of Surgery
Wake Forest University School of Medicine
Chief of Surgery Wake Health
Winston-Salem, NC, USA

Preface

Managing a trauma center is the most difficult role a surgeon can play. It involves complex clinical care, long nights and days, administrative work, self-examination, and critical review of patient care and significant regulatory requirements. There are excellent textbooks available that address prehospital, emergency department, ICU, operating room, and hospital care of the injured but no text that describes clinical issues, administrative processes, performance improvement, and site visit preparation in one work.

In this book, I have attempted to provide key information on all aspects of trauma center management. This knowledge comes from 25 years as a director of a Level 1 trauma center and over 150 inspections of trauma centers across the country.

Any of the chapters or sections of this work can be read independently; however, a physician thinking about leading a trauma center should read as much of the entire book as possible since it will help them understand the enormity of responsibility they will be taking on in that role.

Charlottesville, VA, USA   Jeffrey S. Young, MD, MBA

Acknowledgments

I would like to thank Kathy Butler, Michelle Pomphrey, Sera Downing, Val Quick, Shannon Critzer, Avis Brent, Amy Bunts, and Forrest Calland for their untiring assistance with running a trauma center. But most importantly, I would like to thank my wife, Denise, and my children, Andy, Steven, Brian, Erin, Leigh, Yogi, Butter, and Decimus, for their support and love.

Contents

About the Author

Dr. Young was born in Brooklyn, New York. He attended the University of Virginia, Medical College of Virginia, and trained in trauma and general surgery at Wake Forest University under the mentorship of Dr. J. Wayne Meredith. He assumed the role of trauma director of the University of Virginia (UVA) Trauma Center in July 1994 and has held that role since.

He is a former member of the National Committee on Trauma, associate chief of staff, chief quality officer, and chief patient safety officer. Currently, he is medical director of the Surgical Subspecialties Service Line at the UVA and is a regional chief for the American College of Surgeons (ACS) Committee on Trauma (COT). He has published over 90 peer-reviewed articles on trauma care and is a tenured professor of Surgery and division chief of Acute Care Surgery. He has been a member of the ACS COT Verification Review Committee since 1998 and has performed over 150 trauma center site visits for the ACS, as well as for the States of Maryland and Oregon.

His wife, Denise, is an associate professor of Obstetrics and Gynecology. He has five children and three dogs. Andy is a general surgery resident, while Steven is a third-year medical student both at the UVA. Brian is a student at James Madison University (JMU) and a paramedic. His daughters, Erin and Leigh, are a freshman at JMU and a high school student, respectively. He lives in Troy, Virginia.

Abbreviations

ABC	Airway, breathing and circulation
ACS	American College of Surgeons
COT	Committee on Trauma
CT	Computed tomography
EAST	Eastern Association for the Surgery of Trauma
ED	Emergency department
EMT	Emergency medical technician
GCS	Glasgow coma scale
GSW	Gunshot wound
ICU	Intensive care unit
IEP	Internal education program
LMA	Laryngeal mask airway
M&M	Morbidity and mortality conference
MDPI	Multidisciplinary Performance Improvement Committee
MRI	Magnetic resonance imaging
MTP	Massive transfusion protocol
OFI	Opportunity for improvement
PI	Performance improvement
POS	Probability of survival
PRQ	Pre-review questionnaire
SICU	Surgical intensive care unit
STN	Society of trauma nurses
TMD	Trauma medical director
TOPIC	Trauma outcomes and performance improvement course
TPM	Trauma program manager
TQIP	Trauma quality improvement project

Introduction

What is a trauma center? In essence, it is a virtual clinical structure comprised of all the core units of a hospital, with a group of dedicated clinicians as the heart and soul of the system. I became interested in trauma care early in life, and in a clichéd fashion, it was from the TV show *Emergency*. For many of us growing up in the 1970s that show introduced us to what appeared to be real-life lifesaving. To be honest, Kelly Brackett, MD, FACS, was my idea of a true physician, so like him, I became a surgeon who spent a lot of time in the emergency department.

My overall background is somewhat unique. My first exposure to patient care was as an emergency medical technician (EMT) in Albemarle County, Virginia, in 1981. I began as an EMT and finished as a cardiac technician, the 1980s equivalent to the current EMT-Intermediate. I finished college and medical school and a general surgery residency and trauma fellowship at Wake Forest Baptist Hospital under the mentorship of J. Wayne Meredith, MD, one of the finest trauma surgeons and men I have had the good fortune to know well. When I left residency, I began my career as the trauma director at the University of Virginia and have remained in that position since 1994.

This book is my attempt to put into words my experiences as a director of a university Level I trauma center. Running a trauma center is a unique vocation in clinical medicine, in that I do many things that the average physician would have no interest in. This includes a plethora of meetings, working with many other physicians to create a consistent model of care and spending a great deal of time criticizing the care we provide. However, unlike many physicians, I spend most of my clinical time saving the lives of people who started out their days never imagining they would need our services.

As a warning, 99% of this book will apply to the characteristics of US Level I and II centers. This is due to the fact that I have spent 25 years running a Level I center. Importantly, I have been a site reviewer for the American College of Surgeon and have inspected over 150 other Level I and II centers in the United States. My experience with Level III centers is sparse; thus, I don't feel I have the knowledge and experience to discuss how they are administered. But many of the general concepts I will discuss apply to all centers.

While this book could have been a collaborative effort, I learned long ago that asking people to help with a project only makes it ten times harder and bugging friends to hand in chapters is not especially pleasant. So all the words written are my own, though dozens of people were instrumental in getting the results we have achieved.

You can read any chapter and hopefully gain some useful information. I have provided several case studies to help illustrate the principles I outline in the chapters. In addition, I have included some documents and tools we use at the University of Virginia Trauma Center or have provided links so that the reader can download the materials.

I thank you for taking the time to read this, and I hope it will help you and your patients.

Three Parts: Structure, Function (Operations), and Performance Improvement

As a wise person once said, outcomes follow structure and structure controls processes. When you are designing a system to provide complex care any time of the day or night, with the possibility of inexperienced clinicians, a strong internal cognitive and organizational structure is essential. Trauma centers lead the medical world in creating these structures to keep care "between the lines" no matter who showed up at your bedside.

To design a functioning trauma system, you need to include all facets: EMS, ED, OR, ICU, acute care, and rehabilitation. In addition, you need a well-functioning outpatient clinic component and an injury prevention and outreach program. No Level I trauma center survives without transfers from other trauma centers and non-trauma centers (non-designated hospitals); thus, a strong relationship with referring hospitals is essential. This can be difficult when, as you improve, your tolerance for substandard care in the periphery decreases, but you need to be supportive and constructive with all criticism.

In this part of the book, we will discuss the structure of a trauma center, its fundamental processes, responsibilities of its key staff, and many other topics.

Part I
Structure

Chapter 1
What Is a Trauma Center?

A trauma center is a hospital devoted to trauma care. At its most basic, it includes a trauma service where seriously injured trauma patients are cared for using guidelines and protocols and an administrative structure. When one of these components is substandard, it will be nearly impossible for the care to be consistent and high quality. I believe a trauma center without guidelines is rudderless. As Brent James at Intermountain Healthcare once taught me, a guideline is merely a tool to measure variation; if you don't have any such tool, then your care is random and variable, depending on the whims of whatever practitioner is in charge. At a trauma surgery meeting in the 1990s, this need for standardization was explained with this analogy. If you have a great chili recipe, and even though you've made it hundreds of times, when you don't use the recipe, it just doesn't come out right and is different every time.

A trauma center is not a place or a location; it is, in essence, a group of professionals devoted to providing optimal care to the injured patient who are also devoted to examining the care they provide and constantly improving it. There are different types of trauma centers: Level I, Level II, Level III, and in some states Level IV. What holds all of these trauma

© Springer Nature Switzerland AG 2020
J. S. Young, *Trauma Centers*,
https://doi.org/10.1007/978-3-030-34607-2_1

center levels together is that they all want to provide good care and they all are constantly looking at improving the care they deliver.

I am often asked if I enjoy being an emergency room doctor. I smile and say that I'm a surgeon who spends time in the emergency room. Some of my best friends are emergency room doctors, but a trauma center does not revolve around the emergency room. In fact the average trauma service patient spends the smallest percentage of time from their admission in the emergency room. The trauma center revolves around the people and processes that are put in place to ensure that injuries are identified and treated quickly. Trauma centers also have a higher bar with regard to the care that they provide. The community expects them to provide organized efficient care and to realize when the patient's needs have exceeded their capabilities and to rapidly transfer that patient to a center that can give the patient optimal care and the greatest chance for a good outcome.

Does Your Community/City Need a Trauma Center?

This is an ongoing area of controversy in the USA and abroad. Unfortunately the desire to create a trauma center usually depends much more on economics than on patient need. Many cities were more than happy to let one university hospital admit 5000 trauma patients a year with little or no help from perfectly capable surrounding hospitals, until reimbursement for trauma improved. At that point, suddenly these hospitals have an interest in trauma care. Regardless of the reason, many of these new players do a good job with injured patients, often because they hire accomplished trauma directors and program managers from established centers. The worry is that as soon as the money disappears, so will the desire to take care of trauma patients.

The usual calculation (only moderately scientific) is that there are 1000 critically injured trauma patients per million of population. This is not always true due to variations in geography, the willingness of certain populations for high-risk behaviors, and such. In my own center, though we only cover approximately 600,000 lives, we see between 1800 and 2000 total patients. But the calculation works relatively well for us since we see about 500 ISS > 15 patients/year.

It is generally accepted that a Level I trauma center should see at least 1200 admissions/year with at least 250 patients with an ISS > 15. This does not mean that a center seeing less patients cannot provide great care; it is merely a framework the American College of Surgeons (ACS) uses to examine trauma centers [1].

Trauma centers require a great deal of commitment. First of all for the general surgeon who specializes in trauma, most of the patients do not require his operating room skills. This often turns many surgeons away from trauma because they do not wish to practice in a non-operative specialty. However in my case over the 25 years of my career, while I wish I could've been in the operating room more regularly, the times I do get to the operating room, I am usually doing lifesaving procedures. While I certainly do not want a surgeon who only gets their ego gratification in the operating room to go into trauma, I do want students and physicians interested in caring for the injured to understand that taking care of the trauma patient involves working in many different parts of the hospital and working with many clinicians and administrators to carry out your job well. I say all this to exemplify that devoting your institution to becoming a trauma center is a difficult decision. Many centers become trauma centers for a short period of time and then give up, and many centers stay in the trauma business long after the enthusiasm for providing care for the injured has waned. It is very difficult to run a trauma center when only hospital administration wants it to happen, and it is very difficult to provide optimal care when only the physicians want to provide care to the injured. Thus the decision on whether your community can support a trauma center depends on not only the population but the attitude of your hospital toward an endeavor that may cause financial losses and which can be extremely frustrating. But for those centers that devote themselves to providing optimal care to the injured, I believe the vast majority find it to be personally rewarding and beneficial to their community.

The ACS provides a consultation service and verification to hospitals that are considering becoming trauma centers (https://www.facs.org/quality-programs/trauma/tqp/center-programs/vrc/process). I would greatly encourage all trauma centers to attain ACS trauma center verification since it is a national standard and is fair and well administered. The consultative visit can prevent frustration down the road when an actual site visit occurs, and it will allow everyone to know what the true expectations are of a trauma center so that they can devote the necessary resources. In the USA every major metropolitan area is covered by trauma centers, yet many rural areas are poorly covered. It is a paradox in that while these rural areas may require optimal trauma care the most, due to long transport times and the dearth of qualified providers, they are the most sparsely served because trauma volumes may be low, and it is difficult to recruit the necessary clinicians to provide great trauma care. Aeromedical resources allow regional trauma centers to care for many rural trauma patients, and my own trauma center covers an area of approximately 22,000 mi.[2] and a population of between 600,000 and 800,000 people depending on how you calculate the census. This provides us with yearly admissions of approximately 1800 patients with between 400 and 500 severely injured patients every year. My service admits over 1000 patients a year of which 70% spend time some time in the intensive care unit. This provides a solid number of clinical cases for our clinicians to maintain competence in all facets of trauma care.

Creating a trauma center is also a political decision for any medical center with their community and their clinical staff. Few large cities are underserved with trauma centers, and few rural states or cities have an overabundance. But most new trauma centers are opened in urban areas, with little or no improvement in trauma center coverage in rural America. There are financial reasons for this, but practically, smaller rural areas have less potential trauma patients; there will not be a sufficient volume of trauma patients to support a full-time trauma surgery practice. There are also long-standing relationships with general surgeons, who are for the most part in private practice environments, who are not enthusiastic about meeting the higher standard required to be verified as a trauma center, and who may be resistant to the hospital hiring a group of surgeons to practice trauma and to potentially provide subsidized competition. But in spite of these obstacles, many highly dedicated trauma surgeons, administrators, and nurses create high-performing trauma centers in community hospitals and rural environments. But the work required to do this effectively should not be underestimated.

Another issue is the level of trauma center that is the goal. As I will describe in later chapters, many hospitals want the cachet associated with being a trauma center and more specifically a Level 1 center. In general, Level 1 centers are differentiated from Level 2s by research and graduate medical education. Level 2 centers are also allowed to transfer out patients that should not ever be transferred out of a Level 1. But since most people strive to be "number 1!", centers that do perfectly good work as Level 3 and Level 2 centers want to move up, but often do not have the infrastructure, clinicians, or commitment to make this jump. Also, the elevation to a higher level may be meaningless to the actual clinical care provided (though in some instances, striving for a higher level can improve clinical performance through greater commitment and resources).

I have seen centers go through contortions to try to meet the criteria for Level 1 designation including creating residencies, paying for relationships with academic centers to have residents rotate, paying for expensive locum tenens contracts, and pushing their facilities to a place they should not go. During site visits, it is usually fairly obvious when a center levelling up is being pushed by a faction, instead of an overall drive to provide a higher level of trauma care. It is rare that any center will meet a higher-level criterion unless the majority of the clinicians and administrators are 100% behind the effort.

In some cities, emergency medical services (EMS) will not transport a patient to a non-designated center, thus providing strong impetus for a hospital to be part of the system. But this can be difficult because these non-designated hospitals will receive virtually no trauma patients until they hold themselves out as a trauma center. Though almost all states will only provisionally verify centers with no track record of care of the injured, this is usually opaque to the community who do not realize that the new center may still be beginning their journey to optimal care, while the long-standing trauma center across town is much farther along in that journey.

Does this mean all non-designated centers provide poor care to injured patients? It does not. There are some centers that can self-motivate to provide acceptable care to the injured. But the lack of a performance improvement program, outside examination of performance through site visits, and standards to follow makes this very difficult. I would advise any center that is caring for a significant number of critically injured patients without designation to be able to explain why they don't feel they can succeed in a verification effort and why. Citizens deserve to get the best care possible in their community of region, and it is my opinion that state and national trauma center designation processes provide the best method available to insure optimal care.

It is vitally important that any facility looking toward trauma center designation should do an insightful examination of the care they provide, their resources, their capabilities, and whether holding themselves out as experts in trauma care is safe and cost-effective. It is also very important to look at the trauma capabilities in their catchment area. Competing trauma centers in areas where the population cannot fully support two centers is becoming more and more common in the USA. This tends to dilute the experience necessary to provide optimal care and may or may not actually improve care of the injured in that community. Your own community must look at the capabilities of its hospital facilities, its population, its EMS resources, and its regional resources, before making the critical decision to support the development of a trauma center. It is virtually impossible for a hospital to become designated without the support of all services, units, clinicians, and administrators that will interact with the injured.

Reference

1. Committee on Trauma, American College of Surgeons. Resource for optimal care of the injured patient. 2014. https://www.facs.org/-/media/files/quality-programs/trauma/vrc-resources/resources-for-optimal-care.ashx?la=en.

Chapter 2
Key Components
of a Trauma Center

Before we discuss the roles of leadership in a trauma center and clinical services, we will discuss the key clinical processes and capabilities that differentiate a trauma center from a non-designated hospital (NDH). Some NDH may have some of these capabilities, but in general many do not because they are rarely needed. The essence of a trauma center is 24/7/365 preparedness for whatever type of injured patient comes through the door, and these clinical components are the keys to saving the critically injured. The American College of Surgeons Optimal Resources document provides information on all criteria for all levels of trauma center [1].

Rapid Emergency Department Evaluation

Almost all critically injured patients enter the hospital through the emergency department. Due to improvements in trauma care nationally, it is becoming less common for patients to stay at NDHs for an extended period before transfers. Most trauma patients either come directly from the scene by ground or air or are taken to the closest hospital where they are evaluated and stabilized by the emergency

© Springer Nature Switzerland AG 2020
J. S. Young, *Trauma Centers*,
https://doi.org/10.1007/978-3-030-34607-2_2

department (ED) staff before transfer to the trauma center. It is often this time spent in non-trauma center EDs that can cause significant harm. On the other hand, some non-trauma center EDs provide lifesaving stabilization, and many patients would not reach the trauma center alive if intubation, chest tubes, or blood transfusion were not initiated at these emergency departments.

But trauma center emergency departments differentiate by:

- A regimented activation system to initiate a team response in advance of arrival
- Nurses and technicians that are familiar with trauma care and resuscitation and are able to rapidly set up a trauma bay and provide all necessary care to the injured patient. They also must be competent in safely transporting critically ill patients throughout the hospital for studies and procedures
- Ability to deliver blood transfusions rapidly, obtain IV access in patients with depleted intravascular volumes, and assist with central line and chest tube placement
- Competent with complex airway management up to and including surgical airway placement
- Ability to rapidly adapt to patients with multiple priorities and needs
- Social workers and chaplains to calm and work with families who are in the middle of the worst day of their life
- Ability to ramp up their systems to accommodate multiple critically injured patients when needed

To meet these competencies, trauma center EDs require nurses who work in the trauma bay to be experienced, have additional in-service training, obtain national trauma nursing certifications and/or training, and regularly restrict their clinical duties to the trauma patient and resuscitation area. These are often the most experienced technicians and nurses in the ED. They will need to be cross-trained in many critical care processes such as arterial lines, chest tubes, large bore venous cannulas, spinal immobilization, and competence with invasive hemodynamic monitoring. They need to be facile with medication administration for intubation, deep sedation, pain control, anxiety control, and blood and blood product administration. The technicians and nurses must possess excellent skills in IV insertion as well.

Immediate Blood Availability

Though virtually all hospitals administer blood and blood products, trauma centers must possess the ability to provide many units of blood immediately to resuscitate hypotensive injured patients. The logistics involved in being able to provide immediately availability of large amounts of blood products can be complex and daunting. Close interaction and cooperation with blood bank personnel is critical.

All trauma centers verified by the American College of Surgeons (ACS) must have a massive transfusion protocol. This process insures that blood is immediately available 24/7/365, that it can be rapidly transported to the patient's bedside, that it escalates as the patient's needs escalate, and that an effort is made to insure that bloods products are not wasted unnecessarily.

My mentor would say that a Level 1 trauma center should be able to "transfuse ten units of blood in 10 minutes within 10 minutes of knowing you need it." To do this, you must have large bore IV access, rapid fluid infusion devices, blood warming devices, and enough personnel to check all blood products and hang them rapidly. Since transfusion reactions can be fatal, the system must insure that care is taken to insure that either universal donor blood is given or if cross-matched blood is given that the blood goes through the same double and triple checks that are done in normal circumstances. Giving a critically injured unstable trauma patient a transfusion reaction is almost universally fatal.

Hospitals with cardiac surgery and/or transplant programs have a head start on this process since these specialties often require massive transfusion. However in those specialties, the need for blood products is usually anticipated, where that is almost never the case in trauma.

Immediate Surgical Response and Availability

Trauma centers must have the capability to take a patient to the operating room immediately 24/7/365. For ACS verified Level 1 and 2 centers, this requires a surgical team (nurse and scrub technician or two nurses) in-house 24/7 and immediate anesthesia availability [1]. While this is not terribly difficult in the middle of the night, it is actually extremely difficult at 8 AM on a weekday. This is because most US operating rooms start their first case at 7:30 AM; thus at 8 AM all rooms may be occupied by patients who have now been put under anesthesia, and even if there is a very short case, at this point an occupied operating room usually cannot be cleared for at least an hour, which is not acceptable. While many centers hold an operating room open and staffed at all times, this can waste a valuable resource most of the day. What many centers do is stagger their start time so there is always an operating room available first thing in the AM, and then a short duration case will become available within 10 minutes of the staggered room start.

Trauma centers cannot possibly be ready for every eventuality (five gunshot wound patients showing up simultaneously), but it is required that they have one room immediately available, and that when that room is in use, a second team must be made ready. Some centers have two teams in-house 24/7 but this is unusual.

In addition to the OR staff and anesthesia, pharmacy resources and surgical attendant staff also need to be ready. A trauma center must have a general/trauma surgeon able to respond to the patient's bedside within 15 minutes of notification 80% of the time. Most Level 1 and many Level 2 centers have a surgeon in-house at all times. There also must be another general surgeon on backup (usually from home) at all times ready to come into the hospital should they be needed.

Radiological Availability and Capability

Imaging is critical to the optimal care of injured patients. Other than a patient with a knife sticking out of the abdomen, or neck, there are few other instances where an injured patient will be taken for definitive treatment without imaging (and a chest x-ray will usually be done even in these cases). A chest x-ray is obtained in the trauma bay in all patients. A pelvis x-ray is often obtained, but more centers are deferring this in stable patients to the more accurate evaluation of the pelvis available on CT scanning.

Ultrasound is used on almost all trauma patients to look for fluid in the abdomen. To do this with reasonable accuracy, the trauma surgeons and emergency physicians will need to undergo training and auditing of performance. Inaccurate interpretation of ultrasound (FAST) in the injured can lead to unnecessary operations or fatal delays in intervention.

CT scanning is done in almost all blunt trauma patients. This process is often referred to as "pan-scanning" and usually involves a non-contrast head CT, cervical spine CT, chest CT with contrast, and abdominal/pelvis CT with IV contrast. From these studies the spine can be imaged through reconstruction of the images avoided further spine imaging in most cases. These scans can usually be completed in ~20–30 minutes, provide information about all body cavities, and have a very high degree of accuracy in identifying life-threatening injuries. Competent and rapid interpretation of CT imaging is critical. Even though many trauma surgeons are able to grossly interpret abdominal CT scans, radiologists are necessary for a high degree of confidence in all interpretations. The number of hospitals with 24/7 in-house radiology attendings is increasing, but many hospitals either rely on interpretation by radiologists from home, teleradiology services, or radiology residents. All trauma centers have to perform performance improvement on radiologic interpretation and response.

Interventional radiology (IR) is being increasingly used in the care of injured patients and has saved many lives that surgery could not. All Level 1 and 2 centers must have IR capabilities and be able to begin assembling a team within 30 minutes of activation.

Rapid Specialty Consultation

Trauma patients require services from multiple specialties on a routine bases. Orthopedics is the most commonly consulted service, but neurosurgery, plastics, and otolaryngology (ENT) all play significant roles in subsets of patients. In addition, medical specialties are regularly required to assist with care of patients with extensive comorbidities and medical complications such as renal failure.

Contrary to the relaxed mode of consultation in routine practice, trauma emergency consultation is entirely different. Orthopedic surgeons regularly must respond to the ED to straighten and splint limbs to allow for CT scanning, along with relocation of joints and care of massive combined wounds. Neurosurgical emergencies are perhaps the most time-sensitive in trauma surgery as "time = brain" in cases with expanding intracranial mass lesions causing shift in the brain and eventual herniation. Complex airway issues can also require emergent consultation from ENT.

Rapid consultation is also essential to allow the trauma surgeon to properly prioritize injuries and treatments. Every trauma surgeon has experienced disjointed care when specialty care plans are changed and the course of the patient is disrupted. Many private practice surgical specialists heroically support trauma centers with rapid and professional response to a call; however, many centers deal with unenthusiastic specialty response, especially for non-operative conditions.

A trauma center monitors and insures adequate specialty response. A delayed response that harms a patient should be dealt with rapidly and if repeated should result in the removal of the surgeon from trauma call. With specialties with manpower issues, such as neurosurgery, there are often only two to three neurosurgeons serving a trauma center, and the demands for a primary and backup neurosurgeon (as required by the ACS) can result in physicians burning out and moving to other jobs when they are consistently on call every 2 of 3 days at a trauma center.

This is where many hospitals fall short in hospital commitment to trauma care. No one can expect a surgical specialist to be available 24/7 and have a busy elective practice to make a living. So it is routine that surgical specialists are compensated for call, and there is often hospital financial support for these departments to allow hiring to decompress call responsibilities.

Critical Care

Almost 50% of admitted injured patients spend some time in the intensive care unit (ICU). In trauma centers the trauma surgeon is expected to maintain overall control of these patients, though critical care physicians can provide services to their patients. Most, if not all, trauma surgeons provide critical care, and many programs supplement the trauma surgeons with pulmonologists and anesthesiologists to provide 24/7 coverage. Trauma critical care is its own discipline, and an experienced medical pulmonology intensivist would not possess the necessary knowledge to care for critically injured patients by themselves. Trauma surgeons will always need to be intimately involved with their ICU patient to prioritize interventions and make other critical decisions.

Critically ill trauma patients are usually housed in a surgical intensive care unit (SICU) along with other types of surgical ICU patients such as general surgery, vascular, and transplant. Staffing should be adequate to insure that an experienced intensivist is available for rapid consultation 24/7, and this role is often filled by the in-house trauma surgeon. The trauma service should participate and lead the performance improvement process on their patients, and this must include the care provided in the SICU.

Rehabilitation and Follow-up Care

Trauma patients often come from varied socioeconomic strata. This can make rehabilitation difficult for the uninsured and underinsured. The trauma center has the responsibility to endeavor to provide trauma patients with occupational therapy, physical therapy, and other service support no matter what their financial status is. Often this requires trauma patients completing their initial therapy as inpatients when transfer to rehabilitation is impossible.

Effective social workers and case managers can improve this process by working closely with families to set up a safe home environment or find rehabilitation opportunities and skilled nursing facilities for their patients.

Reference

1. Committee on Trauma, American College of Surgeons. Resource for optimal care of the injured patient. 2014. https://www.facs.org/-/media/files/quality-programs/trauma/vrc-resources/resources-for-optimal-care.ashx?la=en.

Chapter 3
Areas of Focus

Performance Improvement (PI)

PI is an essential component of all trauma centers, and it plays a much larger role in trauma care than in other clinical efforts. Essentially, all of medicine has been working to catch up with what trauma centers have been doing for decades. A gap that was filled by the trauma quality improvement program (TQIP, https://www.facs.org/quality-programs/trauma/tqp/center-programs/tqip) of the American College of Surgeons was the ability to measure whether outcomes had improved and where your center stood next to other centers.

The general guidelines for the activities of the PI program are in Table 3.1. The ACS refers to these efforts as performance improvement and patient safety. But in this book, we will call this process performance improvement (PI). They are explained in more detail in the PI chapter.

In general trauma centers follow the Plan-Do-Study-Act principles that are core to all PI activities across industries. While different tools may be incorporated (Lean, Six Sigma, etc.), an interesting tool with a catchy name does not substitute for the hard work required in identifying issues (while

© Springer Nature Switzerland AG 2020
J. S. Young, *Trauma Centers*,
https://doi.org/10.1007/978-3-030-34607-2_3

TABLE 3.1 Activities of PI program [1]

Monitor trauma care
Have a comprehensive performance improvement plan
Have a reliable method of data collection
Conduct peer review through specialty liaisons
Carry out multidisciplinary review and system performance review through regular meetings
Reduce unnecessary variation
Prevent adverse events
Integrate with hospital PI

being hard on yourself), having crucial conversations with involved clinicians, developing coherent action plans, and following through. Whatever tool you use, these actions must be carried out in a timely fashion.

Financial

As in most hospital-based systems run by clinicians, financial information is often only forthcoming if it is bad news. Whether you are successful or not, trauma center leadership should endeavor to be informed about the financial performance of their patient population. While this is not a requirement for verification, it is important for the survival of the program. As we found out after obtaining this information, the trauma center's patients were providing a margin equal to or exceeding that of any group other than the most profitable and were certainly not operating at a loss when reimbursement versus costs were examined [2]. Many centers prefer to report the trauma patients' performance in relation to charges, which as most of us know will always indicate losses since the charge figure is often an optimistic fantasy.

Since we cannot control the financial status of our patients, our only mechanism to improve financial performance is to control costs. In this area, we need to be careful. An instance where $1000 is saved by not obtaining a CT scan in a patient with a high risk mechanism can come back to haunt the center financially should the patient have a serious undiagnosed injury. In our center, our aggressive stance toward a complete workup for traumatic injury has been accepted by the vast majority of clinicians as the safest and most cost-effective process. This acceptance comes from the examination of the cost and time invested in patient complaints when they are sent home with undiagnosed and untreated injuries and in the increased costs of care resulting from their subsequent delayed treatment, regardless of whether they choose to pursue a malpractice action.

This does not mean that everyone receives a head, cervical spine, chest, abdomen, and pelvic CT scan (pan-scanning). It means that you create an organized, evidence-based guideline for the workup of the injured that uses science and not gut feeling to determine what tests should be obtained.

Another financial wildcard is physician charges. It is difficult to obtain physician costs since this cannot be measured accurately. We found that our patients were appearing to be overall losses because certain specialist charges were very high. This would often create MD charges in excess of the entire charges for a 10-day inpatient stay. There is no easy answer to this, other than to separate out these charges and examine them separate from controllable charges.

Liaisons

Most trauma patients require specialist care; this is a simple fact. A trauma center that has a strong general surgical component but weak specialty collaboration is going to be a weak center. While orthopedics may be considered the key specialty association, neurosurgery, anesthesia, and emergency medicine are all essential partners in optimal trauma care. As we talk about performance improvement, we will touch on problems that occur with specialty collaboration and will describe ways to make strong collaborations.

In essence, the liaisons are required to participate in guideline protocol creation and performance improvement and are required to be the point person to bring back to their faculty issues related to adverse events and physician performance. A weak specialty liaison will allow problems to fester and will increase anxiety and confrontations between services. A strong specialty liaison works as a partner with the trauma center administrative staff trauma care. Exceptional liaisons also can help with EMS and trauma system issues and can raise the bar for patient care throughout an entire region.

Physicians

Other physicians who care for trauma patients must be brought into the philosophy and practice of the trauma center. One saying that I often use is "improvising is good for jazz, but not good for patient care." When physicians violate policy and create their own standard work for the care they provide, this breeds confusion, anxiety, and conflict between nurses and physicians and between physicians. This is why it is vital that the trauma center administration work to make care all-inclusive and have an ironclad system for distributing information to all physicians who may encounter a trauma patient. It should be an expectation that care is consistent and variability only occurs when absolutely necessary. What we often say in our center is that we want to improve and we want to change our protocols and guidelines if they are not in the best interest of the patient. But we have a mature evidence-based discussion about this and will not be improvising protocols on the fly, in the middle of the night.

A solid forum for communicating with all care providers is an essential component of a solid trauma system. This can be accomplished by having key specialty representatives invited to PI activities, publishing a newsletter, giving grand rounds to other departments, etc.

Nurses

Nursing care is the core of good patient care. It is vitally important that your trauma program manager work well with nurses in many clinical areas. It will be the nursing administration that will often have to investigate, analyze, and set up corrective actions among nursing units. The nursing relationships must be collaborative and should be friendly. When you have a nursing staff that is involved and willing to improve the care of the injured patient, you are in good shape. When you have a nursing staff that is disconnected and unenthusiastic about the care of the injured, you have problems.

Emergency Department

The emergency department is the portal for entry for most trauma patients. It is also vital for the trauma center administration to realize that they only see a small percentage of the patients that an emergency medicine physician sees in an average day. Therefore they must be sensitive to the fact that an emergency medicine physician is often trying to triage among five minimally injured patients and one severely injured patient. You should stress to them that it is your job to make their life easier and to take over the care of the severely injured rapidly and efficiently to allow them to continue their job of controlling their emergency department. A trauma team disrupts an emergency department when they are loud, rude, and inefficient. The trauma director's role in creating a seamless efficient system for the care of the injured requires collaboration with emergency physicians. This does not mean that the trauma center gives control of the care of the severely injured to emergency physicians; rather it means that the trauma center administration works together with the emergency department (both the nurses and the physicians) to ensure that triage is appropriate, consultation and activation are timely, and the care is provided as a team. We will look further at this in subsequent chapters.

EMS

I personally have a strong relationship with emergency medical services. I spent my college years as a medic with several EMS agencies and have spent the last 5 years as an operational medical director to three agencies. I've also had experience with the state administration of EMS services as well. Obviously EMS is a critical component to optimal care of the injured patient. However EMS care can be far more variable than inpatient care and can involve municipal politics and regional conflict. In our center, we stress the use of our aeromedical support as our tool for influencing EMS care throughout our region. I also strongly recommend the trauma center administration participate in our local emergency medical services regional boards and performance improvement councils. You must share information with your local EMS agencies, and you must solicit them for comments regarding the ease of transfer of injured patients and the professionalism of your staff when they interact with EMS. Though there is great controversy about the proper role of advanced life support in the seriously injured, stressing airway control, ABCs, and rapid transport to the most appropriate center are the key components of a strong trauma – EMS system.

Relations with Rest of Hospital

Trauma care does not occur in a vacuum. As you ramp up to provide world-class trauma care, you will be using radiology services, laboratory services, transportation, blood bank, rehabilitation, operating room, critical care, and acute care services for a variable number of patients every day with often intense psychosocial needs. While you must be a strong advocate for the needs of the injured patient, you must also be cognizant that these services and resources are also needed by other patients. You can advocate for the care of the injured while also being sensitive to the fact that you cannot monopolize resources and activate them unnecessarily. This requires a strong relationship with the staff of all these areas and with the physician and nursing leaders.

I like to make a special mention of the operating room as the main service that often demands immediate and highly complex teamwork. Saving critically injured patients' lives that require immediate operative intervention cannot really go on anywhere other than the operating room. One of my better-known quotes in my center is that "procedures can be done in the emergency department but operations should be done in the operating room." A chest tube is a procedure; a thoracotomy with lung resection is an operation. So we often require the operating room to set up a room with nurses and anesthesia available all with about 10 minutes warning. There are patients where operative intervention is needed with 30 minutes to preserve their life. To do this effectively, your activation system should insure that the OR is notified immediately about a potential operative patient. You need to develop a system where the OR is notified very early, but not unnecessarily. You also must deactivate the OR as soon as possible if it is apparent that the patient will not need their services. This is a key element, since an operating room that discerns that you do not care about their resource utilization will become uncooperative.

References

1. Committee on Trauma, American College of Surgeons. Resource for optimal care of the injured patient. 2014. https://www.facs.org/-/media/files/quality-programs/trauma/vrc-resources/resources-for-optimal-care.ashx?la=en.
2. Young JS, Cephas GA, Blow O. Outcome and cost of trauma among the elderly: a real-life model of a single-payer reimbursement system. J Trauma. 1998;45:800–4.

Chapter 4
Trauma Center Organizational Structure

Structure follows function and vice versa. If the structure of your trauma center does not optimally support the functions of the various services, your trauma care will be inefficient and unorganized. If the structure of your center supports these functions, then good care should be seamless and, while not effortless, should not be a consistently difficult process.

Patient Care Units and Clinical Services

The key component of the trauma center is the trauma service. The trauma service is usually administered by the trauma director and the core group of trauma surgeons. In Level I trauma centers, the trauma service is usually administered by physicians who devote their clinical career to trauma and critical care. One thing that truly separates the emergency medicine physician and the trauma surgeon is the fact that emergency medicine physician's practice includes critical care only a minority of the time, often with the bedside assistance of inpatient critical care specialists. A trauma surgeon practices critical care for the majority of their clinical activities. In my experience once trauma patients moved out of the

© Springer Nature Switzerland AG 2020
J. S. Young, *Trauma Centers*,
https://doi.org/10.1007/978-3-030-34607-2_4

intensive care units, their problems mostly relate to physical therapy, occupational therapy, and placement and are rarely life-threatening. Thus, what goes on in the ICU is critical to the survival of trauma patients.

You may be surprised that the emergency department was not listed as the primary clinical unit. This is because for mature trauma centers, the emergency department is mostly a portal for the entrance of injured patients into your trauma center. In mature centers, the trauma service works toward lowering emergency department dwell times. We strive to keep this time under 180 minutes or less for all patients, less than 30 minutes for highest level activations, and less than 90 minutes for lower level activations. The reasons for this are that the emergency department often flexes up and flexes down depending on volume and the amount of clinical resources that can be devoted to the trauma patient can vary widely. The purpose of the emergency department is to conduct the initial resuscitation and diagnostic phase and then transition the patient to CT scan or an interventional unit. We try very hard to not return the patient to the emergency department once they leave to go to radiology.

Other than the emergency department, the key units of the trauma service are the primary critical care unit, the step-down unit, and the acute care floor. The presence of step-down units in American hospitals is variable. In trauma care, different than many other specialties, there is a large subset of patients that benefit from step-down care. These are patients with multiple rib fractures, noncritical spinal cord trauma, minor to moderate head injuries with a small amount of intraparenchymal blood, and many others. These patients are often awake and hemodynamically stable, and placing them consistently in the intensive care unit takes up beds that could be used more effectively for critically ill patients. Thus a step-down unit provides an excellent alternative for this wide subset of patients.

The acute care unit is obviously the penultimate destination for trauma patients before discharge. It is in this unit where the families must come to grips with the effects of injury, is where the patient continues and intensifies their physical and occupational therapy, and is where the decisions are made as to where the patient will be discharged to. This could be home, skilled nursing facility, rehabilitation facility, or some other venue. What may surprise many people is that in my experience trauma patients only begin to have detailed memories of their care once it begins in the acute care unit. Due to the large volume and number of sedatives that are used in the intensive care unit, we often find that patients have absolutely no recollection of the emergency department and intensive care unit phase of care. Thus it is essential that in the acute care unit, the patients and families are deeply supported.

Administrative Leadership

At this point I will discuss in more detail the role of the key administrative leaders of the trauma center. These are the trauma medical director (TMD) and the trauma program manager (TPM). The American College of Surgeons committee on trauma specifies discrete duties for the TMD and TPM. I will go over many of these duties specifically.

Trauma Medical Director

The TMD is the leader of the trauma center. The TMD must be a board-certified or in non-ACS verified centers board eligible general surgeon. It is preferable that the TMD also be subspecialty boarded in critical care medicine and has done a trauma/critical care fellowship, but this is not mandatory. The TMD is the lead person for relationships with the hospital and other services, should lead the PI program and be responsible for loop closure and collaboration with other physician services, and should look out for the financial health of the program and recruitment of new faculty and advanced practice practitioners. In the vast majority of trauma centers, the

TMD is an active trauma surgeon taking their turn in the clinical administration of the inpatient service and taking call, but this is not universal. It is required by the American College of Surgeons that the TMD participate in clinical care of trauma patients, but the amount of time the TMD spends doing that is variable.

The TMD is responsible for the quality of care delivered throughout the trauma center. This is a new concept to many physicians and that they are usually only responsible for the care that they provide. But a competent TMD must view every injured patient that enters the doors of their trauma center as their own patient and must look out for that patient's well-being. In addition the TMD's influence extends beyond the doors of the trauma center to the EMS community and to their state administration of EMS. It is mandatory that the TMD be involved in local regional EMS issues and preferable that they are involved at the state level. This is usually second nature to most TMDs since competent EMS care is essential to optimizing the survival of injured patients. The TMD should also be the lead liaison to other hospitals and to EMS agencies beyond their local catchment area.

I would encourage the reader to look at the "optimal resources for the care of the injured patient" document produced by the American College of Surgeons committee on trauma [1]. This document outlines all requirements for verification for all levels of trauma centers from a national verifying body. I will not reiterate all of the information related to the TMD and TPM that is contained in that document but will try to give specific examples of what the TMD is responsible for in their daily activities.

Who Is the Right Person for Trauma Medical Director?

There are many types of effective trauma medical directors throughout the country. But it is worth discussing what type of physician is best suited to this role. Trauma medical directors can be hired straight out of fellowship but more often are hired midcareer after spending time as trauma faculty in a designated trauma center. I myself was hired right out of fellowship, but I was trained by one of the leading trauma medical directors in the country, and a great deal of my additional year was spent on topics relevant to managing a trauma center. Not all graduates of trauma and critical care fellowships will have that kind of experience.

Trauma medical direction is an active role not a passive role. Even after a quarter-century as a high-performing Level I trauma center, I have to deal with problems and develop and implement corrective action plans at least once or twice a week. This is important in that small problems can become big problems fairly quickly, and as you gain experience as a trauma medical director, interventions and corrective actions come more easily and are more easily implemented. It is vital that a potential trauma medical director can build consensus. A dictatorial style may appear to be effective for a short period of time, but people who are dissatisfied with decisions and who are not given the opportunity to voice their opinion can slowly poison the program from within. It is not essential that there be unanimity in decision-making, but it is essential that people are allowed to express their opinion, and it is incumbent upon the leader to explain their reasoning. It is also vitally important that the trauma medical director gain the respect of clinicians and staff by being active in trauma care. This sets an example for the entire center, and the medical director will quickly lose the respect of the trauma center staff if they are seen as someone who sits in their office issuing edicts. It is optimal that the trauma medical director has a vast and encompassing knowledge of traumatology and be an excellent clinician. Is often difficult to assess a potential candidate's clinical skills during the interview process, but I feel a distinct investigation should be made with the candidate's mentors and faculty in residency and fellowship to get an honest appraisal of their ability to lead clinically.

There are really four types of trauma centers and each requires a certain type of direction:

- A center that provides good care but believes they provide suboptimal care

  - This is probably the highest-performing type of center and that they are constantly looking for ways to improve and not resting on their laurels.

- A center that provides good care and believes they provide good care

  - A center like this is not hurting any patients but may be deficient in performance improvement activities by believing that they are already functioning at the highest level possible.

- A center that provides suboptimal care and believes they provide suboptimal care

  - This is actually the situation I found myself in when I arrived in my current position. You can work with this type of center, and they are anxious about the care they are providing and are looking for leadership. This does not mean that improving a center like this will be easy, but it does mean that you will not have to deal with the obstacles of arrogance and overconfidence.

- A center that provides suboptimal care but believes that they provide great care

  - This is possibly worst position for a trauma medical director. Not only will they have to and improve trauma center performance and patient care but they will also have to overcome arrogance and inaccurate perception of the quality of care. A center such as this will be far better served by an experienced trauma medical director who has already been in that position at another verified trauma center. The best candidate for this would be someone who has reformed another trauma center.

It is important to remember that a trauma medical director that has reformed another trauma center may not be loved by that trauma center. Often leaders are brought in to cause disruption by executive leadership that knows that the center must improve. It is an outstanding individual who can overcome obstacles and still be respected and loved, but unfortunately it is common for directors who have to perform major reconstruction of a center to create bad feelings among those who are satisfied with the status quo.

There are many outstanding trauma critical care fellowships throughout the country; however it is important to note that all but very few concentrate on teaching physicians clinical care. There are only a few trauma fellowships where a significant amount of time is spent on the issues relevant to someone who will go out and be a trauma medical director. So graduating from a fellowship that is known for training outstanding clinicians does not guarantee that the graduating fellow has been taught knowledge and skills necessary to direct the trauma center. In addition many traumatologists across the country have no desire to direct a trauma center, and those people should not be forced into doing so. It is possible with a great deal of support to take someone who was unenthusiastic about being a leader and turn them into an adequate director. But it is probably easier for the process of building or reforming a trauma center to find someone who has both the skills and desire to direct the trauma program. But there are not that many people around, and many of them are employed in centers that they have built and can be reticent to leave. In conclusion the trauma program director cannot be assigned as the one person who didn't attend the meeting where roles were handed out. The director must be enthusiastic in running the center, must be clinically capable, and must be able to be a team player and build consensus among a wide variety of clinicians and administrators.

Organization of Care and the TMD

The TMD is responsible for creating the guidelines that will decrease variability in the care provided to injured patients. The TMD can use guidelines created by national trauma organizations or can develop them themselves. These guidelines should reflect the latest evidence available in the care of injured patients, and it is the TMD's responsibility once they are created to disseminate them to all the physicians and nurses and other providers that may come in contact with injured patients. There are no regulations for the number of guidelines that are created, but at the very least, they should include the initial evaluation resuscitation of the injured patient, triage guidelines, basic ICU guidelines for ventilatory management and fluid/blood resuscitation, massive transfusion protocols, and mandatory consultation guidelines. Our own protocol manual [2] runs over 180 pages and includes virtually every major condition and injury complex. It also includes guidelines for pediatric trauma and burn. This is usually beyond the scope of most online manuals, but the more that you write down, the more it demonstrates that you thought about the care to be delivered for these conditions. In addition, as I said previously, a guideline is merely a tool to measure variation, and without that tool there is no way to measure variation. It is not necessary for the trauma program to audit compliance with all of these guidelines, but it is a very good idea for the program to audit compliance with the most important of these. This is usually a key component of the PI plan for the program for any given year.

The TMD has extensive responsibilities in performance improvement. The TMD is responsible for the creation and the completion of corrective action plans for opportunities for improvement (OFI). Performance improvement programs are not all structured identically, though there should be many common components among them. In some the TMD provides the first level review for many issues, especially deaths, and in others the TPM will provide the first level review and triage problems to the TMD. We will go into this further in the PI chapters. The TMD is responsible for the PI meetings and is also responsible for ensuring that these meetings carry out a thorough analysis and discussion of issues, the corrective action plans are created, they are assigned, due dates are assigned, and these plans are followed to completion. An associate TMD can be the chair of the PI meetings, but the TMD should sign off on all results and attend the meetings at least 50% of the time (hopefully far more often). Organizing the service and being the lead clinician for performance improvement are essentially the two main components of the TMD's job.

Trauma Program Manager

The TPM is a nurse usually with Master's training who is responsible for the administration of the trauma program. The TPM usually oversees the trauma office which will always include the trauma registrar but may also include PI coordinators and other administrative assistants. The TPM is responsible for organizing the PI program and also determines with the TMD what events will be reviewed by the program and what PI projects will be done for the coming year. One of the most important aspects of the TPM's job is preparation for site visit. It is a fact of life for all trauma centers that they are verified and certified by certain agencies. The American College of Surgeons committee on trauma verification review committee provides the largest number of verifications in the country, but many states still have their own homegrown verification systems. However even these local systems are usually based on the materials created by the verification review committee. They may include additional criteria that are important to their state and also may remove certain criteria that they don't feel are relevant. It is the responsibility of the TPM to ensure that the program stays on track with all criteria in their verification regulations and to correct any deficiencies. At the site visit, it is usually the TPM that spends the most time with the site visit team, and thus he or she must be the most knowledgeable about all aspects of the program. We will go into more about site visits and verification in later chapters.

What Type of Person Should Be the Trauma Program Manager?

With the trauma medical director, the trauma program manager is probably the most important part of a well-functioning trauma center. The trauma program manager will often be the effector arm of the trauma leadership. They will direct registry activities and performance improvement. They will also be responsible for evaluations of trauma center staff and will supervise the hiring and firing of employees.

Optimally this person will have served as a trauma program manager in another center, or as an assistant trauma program manager. However it is often impossible to lure a current manager from their center, and the role of assistant trauma program manager varies widely throughout the country.

The trauma program manager must be a registered nurse preferably with a Master's degree with experience in either the emergency department, flight nursing, or critical care. It is preferable that they held a leadership role in those areas.

It is vital that the trauma program manager be an experienced clinician because they will spend a great deal of time working in nursing units educating nurses and ensuring low-variability care for injured patients. In most hospitals with high census, injured patients will often reside on "ectopic" floors where the nurses may not be as familiar with their care. It is often the responsibility of the TPM and their staffs to go and educate these nurses to ensure high-quality, low-variability care for their patients. Thus preparation for site visit, maintaining verification, and being an educational resource to nurses and clinicians are the primary components of the TPM's job.

The Administrative Relationship Between TMD and TPM

The ACS requires that the TMDs have the authority to administer the trauma program. However many hospitals have different administrative structure for nurses and physicians. It is uncommon especially in academic hospitals for physicians to be in complete command of a clinical service (including clinical, administrative, and financial authority). This is usually managed by an administrator with directors and managers below them. Thus meeting the letter of the law for the ACS regarding the TMD's ability to completely administer a program can be difficult. At the very least, the TMD must be involved in the creation of the budget, the performance evaluations of the members of the program, all hiring and firing, and reporting up to the hospital administrative and quality structure. However in many programs, it will be impossible to structure a system where the TPM reports to the TMD. TPMs usually report through nursing administration or hospital administration, and TMDs usually report to the Chief Medical Officer. Because of this variability, a clean reporting structure may be impossible. What the teams will be looking for is the ability of the TMD to remove inadequate personnel from either the administrative or clinical parts of the program, to be successful in gaining approval for key budget items and to be able to work with the TPM to administer the program appropriately. It is optimal if the TPM can report to the TMD, but some hospitals just do not allow this reporting structure.

Physician Leadership (Liaisons)

While the liaison positions are not usually compensated, the performances of these physicians are critical to optimal care. The key liaisons are orthopedics, neurosurgery, emergency medicine, and now radiology and critical care. The liaison should be a senior or at the very least a midcareer board-certified clinician. The liaison is required to attend 50% of all the multidisciplinary PI (MDPI) meetings and to be the lead collaborator between the trauma program and the respective disciplines. It is often the failure of liaison that leads to significant problems and clinical care.

One of the key issues in trauma center management is that though trauma care is usually the most important clinical activity for the TMD, it is rarely the most important clinical activity for the liaison or the clinicians in their departments. Thus the liaison often has the difficult job of creating changes in practice among the disparate group of clinicians who do not view trauma care as their focus. The liaison will often require a great deal of assistance from the TMD and TPM to make change in their departments. This assistance can range from personal involvement to education and provision of evidence to help convince their clinicians to follow guidelines and to decrease variability.

There've been many books written on having crucial conversations and building consensus among professionals, and we will certainly not spend a great deal of time talking about that, but I have learned some things over the years. I am referencing two books that I found most helpful [3, 4]. First it is essential to speak personally to the leader of the liaison's departments to ensure that they will back up the liaison and use their influence to create change. Second, it is essential that the TMD listen when they state that there are clinical conditions that simply do not have overall national consensus or do not have compelling evidence for a guideline. While citizens like to believe that there is evidence for all that we do, there've been many studies to show that only 20–25% of current clinical care practices are supported by evidence from randomized prospective trials or prospective trials of any type. Much of clinical care is based on the "usual" practice and expert opinion. In my opinion, it is important to use outcomes as a way of supporting the liaisons' efforts to change care. If outcomes appear to be suboptimal and there is no clear scientific support for one clinical practice over another, it is not unreasonable to carry out experiments (PI research, meaning you will use the scientific method but for the purpose of improving care, not for publication) to determine the optimal clinical pathway. It is also vital to provide feedback to clinicians concerning the results of PI analysis.

There are specialties that are notorious for being guided by personal preference and not current evidence. It is very difficult as a trauma director to dictate to a specialist how they should provide care if it is outside of general surgery and critical care. It is incumbent upon the liaison to translate the most recent evidence into bedside care. However in many instances there can be significant resistance to adopting new strategies. The trauma director needs to use their ability to build consensus, the most recent literature, and the philosophy of putting the patient first to help guide the center to the most up-to-date specialty care. In addition, as I stated previously, the director needs to be sensitive to the fact that a great deal of clinical care is not supported by high-level evidence. But even in these situations, it is important that clinical conditions are not treated differently every hour of every day of the week. If there is no clear evidence-based way to take care of a certain condition, for the sake of the patient, it is best that the trauma medical director and the liaison try to reach consensus on a consistent method of treatment.

Core Trauma Units and Services

The nursing leaders of your key clinical units are also very important part of your trauma program. You must build good relationships with these nurses, and you must utilize them to help spread clinical knowledge and to encourage their nurses to report problems with the clinical care of the injured. A trauma program built without the support of the key unit managers will almost invariably have a high level of variability and will not have a robust program for identifying opportunities for improvement.

Nurses tend to chafe at the responsibility of policing and enforcing care guidelines. Many do not feel it is their role to report a clinician going off guideline and that this potentially poisons the relationship between that provider and the nurse. This is especially true in academic training programs where residents are very sensitive to criticism. However the nurses are on the front line, and they are the most aware of variation, so that they must be involved in auditing in some way to have a continually improving trauma center.

ED

The ED nursing manager is a key player in your trauma program. They must be part of your MDPI committee and should be close collaborators with your TPM. There are several key issues where the ED nursing manager can play a vital role. First is the creation of criteria and educational programs for the nurses that will work in the trauma bay. This is often a weakness in many programs, and nurse staffing in the emergency department can be extremely variable and have very high turnover. Thus it is difficult to create a core group of nurses to work with the trauma team, and it is also very difficult to ensure that they participate in enough trauma activations to maintain competence and that they gather yearly education to improve their skills and cognitive knowledge. The ED nursing manager is essential for making a strong core group of trauma bay nurses. Second many opportunities for improvement will occur in the emergency department phase, and corrective action plans will often involve significant effort on the part of the ED nursing manager. As in all other relationships, it is essential to not dictate to the nursing manager but collaborate with them to improve care. This process can be slow, but usually dictating to other professionals what they must do is not as effective in moving care forward by developing solutions together so that they can get buy-in from their troops.

Here is an example from my own experience from a Clinicalbraintraining.com podcast:

> When I started as trauma director, the trauma center was a mess. While we had nominally been a trauma center for several years we did not truly have a trauma director. We had a surgeon who had heroically taken that role but who is not clinically active and who could carry out some administrative functions, but could not clinically lead the center. In fact there was a huge blowup over the role of emergency medicine and trauma, with emergency medicine feeling that since nobody on the surgery side was supervising care that they were obligated to take over command for the safety of the patient. One of the first things I had to deal with was the first five minutes when the patient arrived. Because the trauma response from the surgery department was so disorganized the

emergency department felt they were being invaded every time they called the trauma alert. The gaggle of people that would show up would completely dominate a room start yelling throwing things around and basically making a spectacle of themselves. I can tell you that what I did was show up for every trauma activation and be down in the ED every time a trauma patient arrived. In actuality I did this for about five years. Once people saw the not only was I going to take care of these patients but I would take responsibility for what happened to them, then they began to defer some authority to the trauma surgery service. Another thing they came up is that the emergency room nurses did not feel that they had a defined role in these first five minutes. An idea actually came up through the emergency medicine nurse ranks that they wanted to have five minutes alone with the patient once they arrived without any physicians examining or talking to the patient this way they could get their vital signs done without anybody hassling them. Anyone who knows anything about trauma care knows this is simply an impossible request but it did come up because of problems that they were seeing. They were being hip checked out of the way by the team and could not even get close enough to the patient to put a blood pressure cuff on. I was also demanding that we obtain vital signs within the first minute after the patient arrived and the nurses were put in a double bind situation. My solution was to get the key emergency department nurses and myself together in a room to discuss what the state-of-the-art was in the first five minutes of trauma resuscitation. We decided where everybody would be standing and what their individual roles would be. We also limited the number of people that would be in the room during resuscitation and anyone who is around the bed had to have a defined role and had to stand in the appropriate place. Naturally in hospitals there are more things written down that are ever actually done so we did have to prove to them that I would come and maintain order during the activations, which I did. Eventually the nursing teams enjoyed working with the traumas as they became more organized and efficient. [5]

However it is still an ongoing problem for trauma surgeons to deal with emergency rooms feel they are being invaded whenever there is an activation. This can lead to some significant PI problems related to under triage and reluctance to call the trauma team down. Some of my best friends are emergency physicians, and I know they are quite competent with trauma care, but my attitude has been that if I'm going to have to take care of that patient throughout their entire hospital course, I really do need to be in command of their care when they initially arrive. In addition, the ACS expects the trauma surgeon to be in command of highest level activations.

Surgical Intensive Care Unit

The surgical intensive care unit (SICU) is an absolutely key location for the optimal care of injured patients. What happens after the patient arrives in the SICU is vitally important to whether they will go home to their family or not. Dealing with the initial resuscitation, diagnosing and obtaining appropriate consultation for all injuries, triaging necessary operations, and providing stronger critical care are all essential for good outcome. The ICU nurses are a key component of this. The ICU manager is obviously a key leader in ensuring that the nurses are properly educated and experienced in the critical care of injured patients.

A trauma surgeon is required by the ACS to either be director or co-director of the SICU. This exemplifies the importance that the ACS places on surgical input and critical care. The trauma surgeon or TMD should create guidelines for critical care of trauma patients and develop admission criteria for the SICU and the neurological ICU if available. In academic centers, the in-house trauma surgeon is often the intensivist responsible for the SICU at night, and trauma surgeons are almost always on the staff of the SICU as intensivists. In academic programs the trauma program should put processes in place such that small problems do not become life-threatening problems without proper involvement of more senior clinicians. The trauma program should be intimately involved with the investigation of mortality and morbidity in the SICU and should work closely with the SICU team to bring about change and proper corrective actions. It is likely the trauma program is one of the few programs in the hospital that is closely monitoring critical care outcomes. Many SICU directors welcome the involvement of the trauma program. It is imperative in Level I centers and in most Level II centers that the care of injured patients not be turned over to an entirely separate team of clinicians in the SICU. There can be mandatory consults for certain aspects of care (ventilator management), but the multiple and critically injured patient must remain under the care of the trauma service. This differs in pediatric care in that the pediatric intensive care unit is usually closed and run by pediatric intensivists. Regardless the pediatric trauma surgeons must demonstrate that they are intimately involved with all the care that is provided. It is not a valid excuse when presenting a case to the ACS that "another team took care the patient and we were not responsible." It is expected that you will be involved and accountable for the critical care that is provided to trauma patients.

EMS

I am putting EMS in one section here so that EMS providers have one place to look for information and so that they don't find it necessary to read all the other less relevant material. I've lectured and written in some venues about my concerns about some of the structure of EMS in the USA. The wide disparity of experience and training among EMS providers even in the same county can make it extremely difficult to have low-variability high-quality care. However EMS providers as a whole are incredibly diligent dedicated personnel who want to do the right thing for patients, and just like doctors they can let their ego get in the way, and they can resist changes in their traditional methods.

The main difficulty of EMS operations is that experience with major trauma is lacking in many EMS organizations. In a lecture that I gave at a trauma symposium in Cleveland, I stated that on average an individual EMS provider in a 100,000–200,000 person county will see a major trauma patient maybe once a month, whereas these patients are ubiquitous on the trauma service of a Level I center. However in the EMS realm, trauma is a relatively simple condition to treat. It mainly involves rapidly evaluating and triaging the patient, initiating some basic care which can be either BLS or ALS, activating aeromedical when appropriate, and, most importantly, taking the patient to the right hospital. It has been shown in multiple scientific studies that triaging critically injured patients to an inappropriate hospital or to a lower level trauma center, when the difference in time between that transported transport to a level one or two center is minimal (<15 minutes), puts the patient at a disadvantage and impairs survival. It is very difficult for an EMS provider to make a complex transport decision on the spur of the moment without some preplanning. That's why it is vital for the trauma center to go out into their EMS community and draw a map to show where they should take a critical patient. A patient may need to go to a non-designated hospital or Level III trauma center initially, especially when the weather precludes aeromedical transport or the distances are such that it would be unsafe to have the patient in a ground ambulance without evaluation by a physician prior to the transport. But, transferring the patient rapidly and seamlessly to the higher level (I or II) trauma center should be a well planned process. It is also vital that they have good systems for activating aeromedical transport. Many systems place the helicopter on 5-minute standby, and some EMS regions even have the ship on airborne standby, cutting off even more time from request to response. In these systems, the helicopter launches when the first EMS provider comes on the scene and confirms a critical patient. Experienced systems have a good relationship with fire and EMS and create preplanned landing zones to allow the helicopter personnel to get to the scene quickly and evacuate the patient rapidly.

Transport Modes

There are basically two transport modes (or possibly three) an EMS provider can choose from. They can transport the patient in their own ambulance, they can transport the patient by helicopter, or they could meet in ALS transport ambulance in route and bring a medic into their BLS ambulance to provide advanced life support. When I was coming up in EMS in the 1980s, the third option was used very frequently because there was a feeling that ALS added valuable procedures and expertise that could positively impact the patient. It was not surprising that further scientific study demonstrated that in trauma patients, there are few procedures available to the paramedic that compensate for the delay in meeting up with that provider. I do feel there are some instances where ALS is lifesaving. Those are instances with a difficult airway or when an airway cannot be obtained by the BLS provider. However in those situations the time course is extremely short, and delays are often fatal.

Another factor is the experience provided by an experienced medic. Though they may not be able to alter the course of the patient with procedures, they often will pick up cues to the seriousness of the patient's condition and expedite extrication and transport which is often lifesaving.

Basic Prehospital Clinical Issues in Trauma Patients

Airway

I have found that hospital providers are much less comfortable with observing a patient with respiratory distress than EMS providers. Due to the fact that EMS providers are not used to obtaining definitive airways and the fact that they do not see the results of long periods of respiratory distress (respiratory failure, tracheostomy, and occasionally death), they can often feel that simply transporting rapidly with lights and sirens is sufficient treatment to someone and who is having respiratory difficulty. I would say in general this is understandable and is in some way safe when the providers have limited airway experience and little or no experience with rapid sequence intubation. However you will find most emergency medicine physicians, anesthesiologist, and trauma surgeons are far more comfortable having a patient with an endotracheal tube than they are with any other option.

We still find it extremely common in the hospital that supraglottic airways are thought to be suboptimal and are not used in emergency situations, though laryngeal mask airways (LMA) have become far more popular in the operating room and as a rescue airway. However some of us who have EMS experience know that these supraglottic airways can be lifesaving. Therefore we adapted our care to allow them to be used in the hospital. Beyond my trauma center responsibilities, I also think that laryngeal mask airways could be lifesaving in those patients in the hospital who have extremely difficult airways and have tried to convince our resuscitation teams to use them and to stock them.

Shock

Emergency medical services ability to manage shock is limited. This can be a significant detriment to survival when transport times are long, and it is a major factor in the decision for picking the appropriate transport mode. Basically, EMS has crystalloid and dopamine (which should almost never be used for hypovolemia) as their therapies for shock. In general dopamine is not indicated in many EMS protocols for hypovolemic shock and is only indicated for cardiogenic and occasionally septic shock. Most if not all EMS agencies do not have access to blood or plasma but this is evolving. Some sophisticated aeromedical services and the military do have blood and plasma available, but as a general rule, crystalloid is the only fluid available.

In addition EMS does not possess techniques for advanced vascular access other than large bore IV catheters. While some EMS agencies experimented with central and femoral line placement, this is certainly not routine. In addition both these techniques require a fair amount of experience and practice, and attempting to place a central or femoral line once every 6 months is likely not going to be successful. I myself have seen cases where the lines have caused fatal complications when they are placed superior to the inguinal ligament and infuse large amounts of fluid into the retroperitoneum. Interosseous IV placement has become routine and can be lifesaving, but a trauma patient with multiple extremity fractures can present a challenge for this technique. Thus in the patient with hypovolemic shock, EMS is limited to placing large IVs and initiating crystalloid resuscitation. Intravenous placement should not delay transport in the critically injured patient. The lines should be placed while the patient is being extricated or after loading into the ambulance as the unit moves toward definitive care. Another problem is the mounting evidence that crystalloid is a poor volume replacement for trauma patients. It has immunosuppressive properties, and it can also worsen acidosis. Though as long as 70 years ago, plasma was used in the European and Far East theaters of World War II, plasma use in the prehospital setting in the USA is rare. I'm hopeful that research in the next few years will allow us to find a more useful prehospital resuscitation fluid.

Other adjuncts such as MAST trousers have fallen by the wayside and are almost historical at this point. While the Iraq and Afghanistan wars put increased emphasis on the use of tourniquets, there is some evidence presented recently with regard to active shooter incidents that may indicate that civilian use of tourniquets may be less important than they were in the military conflicts. However it is essential that every prehospital vehicle equipped with easy-to-use and effective tourniquets and personnel are well-trained in their use. It is an important role of the trauma center to aid with this education and provide opportunities for EMS providers to learn in a simulated setting. The College of Surgeons "Stop The Bleed" course [6] is simple and can be lifesaving, and every trauma center should be teaching this course and expanding the number of people with training.

Splinting and Immobilization

There is no area with more change in practice in the prehospital realm than in the areas of splinting and immobilization. Both of these areas have undergone tremendous change in just the past 5 years. When I was trained as an EMT in the early 1980s, we were taught extensively in the placement of traction splints and other splints and were taught to try to place limbs in their normal anatomic position in almost all instances. At the present time, EMTs are taught to position extremities as they lay unless there is obvious evidence of neurovascular compromise, and simple straightening to anatomic position should be performed. Other than controlling bleeding with pressure dressings, there is little else that can be done to mangled or injured extremities in the prehospital arena. Two tools that I would like to mention are Israeli combat dressings and hemostatic dressings. I have found both of these products are incredibly useful in the lacerations that are associated with major extremity fractures. The lacerations tend to bleed slowly but extensively over a period of time, and because the bleeding does not appear life-threatening it can often cause significant amounts of blood loss. In several instances I've used the Israeli compression hemostatic dressing over open fracture sites to easily control this bleeding and prevent unneeded blood loss. For deep wounds with significant bleeding, hemostatic gauze can be packed into the wound, and this can be very effective. Trauma surgeons should stress to all prehospital providers to never place two individual pieces of gauze deep in a wound. When clot forms it is very easy to lose a deeply placed gauze dressing, and they can remain to dwell in the wounds and cause infection over time. EMTs should be told to use one long piece of dressing or to tie a knot between two long pieces of dressing to ensure that when you remove the most superficial piece, you will be able to remove the deeper dressing.

Regarding spinal mobilization, there's been tremendous change in the last several years. In the past, great effort was spent in the prehospital area to ensure spinal alignment and to minimize movement for victims of blunt and penetrating trauma. However recent studies have demonstrated that spinal immobilization provides very little overall protection for the cervical or thoracic spine and that in the absence of grossly unstable fractures, they do more harm than good. For those of us that work with EMS closely, we have tried to steer a middle road between not immobilizing anyone and staying with our full immobilization schemes. The conclusion many medical directors have come to is that awake patients without spine pain or tenderness, regardless of mechanism, can move themselves to stretchers where a cervical collar can be secured and the patient can be transported to the hospital without a backboard. We still have a great deal of anxiety over the unconscious patient and feel the full immobilization is still required. However in a boon to many EMS agencies, the practice of immobilizing a patient found to be standing on the scene will hopefully become historical. In addition, full mobilization for victims of penetrating trauma in the absence of clear neurological deficits has been abandoned.

It is vital that the trauma center maintains situational awareness of the EMS protocols that are being put in place in their referring agencies. Trauma centers should be diligent about providing transporting agencies with feedback concerning the patient that they bring in, missed injuries, immobilization deficits, and other problems that can improve the care to injured patients. It is also vital that trauma centers listen to complaints and criticism from EMS providers concerning communication, feedback, handoff of care, and resuscitation room practices. EMS providers must always be thought of as team members of the trauma team.

Operating Room

While the OR is not routinely used by the general trauma surgeons, it is used in well over 50% of trauma admissions. Orthopedic operations tend to dominate, and good OR availability is key to decreasing morbidity through early ambulation and decreasing length of stay. The OR manager or administrator should be part of the PI committee as well as the anesthesiology liaison.

The operating room must be able to staff a room immediately any time of the day or night for a critical trauma patient. This does not mean that a room is left open at all times but that a plan must be in place to create a room rapidly. There are flow studies that demonstrate that if your OR has more than ten rooms, there is always one room that can be made available rapidly. One bad time of day is a weekday when the operating room schedule starts (usually 7:30 AM). At that time of day, it is best for the OR staff to stagger the start in one room and to make certain there is a short case in one of the rooms.

A site reviewer will often ask "what would you do if a gunshot wound to the abdomen with a blood pressure of 60 rolled into your emergency room at 8AM on a Tuesday?" Your OR staff should have a direct answer that involves a well-thought out plan for preparedness at any time of the day and night. We all realize there may be times when it will be difficult several, simultaneous multiple trauma patients to go into operating rooms immediately, but there should be no excuse for not having a room immediately available for one critical trauma patient at all times.

References

1. Committee on Trauma, American College of Surgeons. Resource for optimal care of the injured patient. 2014. https://www.facs.org/-/media/files/quality-programs/trauma/vrc-resources/resources-for-optimal-care.ashx?la=en.
2. Young JS. Spring 2019. https://www.medicalcenter.virginia.edu/intranet/trauma-center/trauma-manual-spring-2019.
3. Grenny J. Influencer. New York: McGraw Hill; 2013.

4. Patterson K. Crucial conversations. New York: McGraw Hill; 2011.
5. Young JS Leadership and improving clinical care. Audio podcast. Clinical Brain Training, Libsyn Publishing; 13 May 2012.
6. Committee on Trauma, American College of Surgeons. 2019. https://www.bleedingcontrol.org/.

Part II
Trauma Center Operations

Chapter 5
Activation Process

Criteria

The criteria for trauma team activation are perhaps one of the most important facets of safe trauma center care. Loose criteria will result in overtriage, and overly tight criteria (or criteria which are ignored) can lead to the late appreciation of life-threatening problems, and unexpected death and disability. Overly inclusive criteria will result in burnout and excess activations will cause conflict with emergency department operations. In general, it is thought that the trauma center should have a 15–30% overtriage rate, meaning that the trauma team should be activated 15–30% more times it is actually needed. This can be difficult to determine; however, two easy analyses of over and undertriage are patients that are admitted to the ICU without a trauma team activation (undertriage) and patient sent home from the emergency department with the trauma team activation (overtriage). These percentages should be measured and viewed by the PI committee at regular intervals.

© Springer Nature Switzerland AG 2020   55
J. S. Young, *Trauma Centers*,
https://doi.org/10.1007/978-3-030-34607-2_5

I will provide you the talking points to explain to your facility why activation criteria are so important and why they need to be fairly broad. First it is been well-established through research, examination of the practices of high-risk industries, and in postmortem examination of disasters that simple systems which bring critical resources to bear rapidly improve outcomes. If you do not gather resources until you find that you are in dire need of them you will delay treatment and intervention every time. I like to call this the "inherent inertia of emergency response."

The "inherent inertia of emergency response" is easy to see. I remember a distinct incident where a patient was coming in with a gunshot wound to the abdomen. This was at a point in our trauma center development where the trauma team was not welcomed into the ED. So the ED felt that we should only be called concurrent with the patient's arrival. Unfortunately, in a case like a gunshot wound, arriving after the patient is already in the trauma bay creates a delay. In addition, there is significant time lost through simple tasks such as moving the patient from the EMS stretcher to the ED bed, completing the initial assessment, obtaining x-rays, and this delay could be as long as 15–20 minutes. Following several incidents like this where I felt the inertia negatively impacted outcomes, I began a policy where for select cases the trauma surgeon would see the patient either on the helipad or in the ambulance bay and, at that point, with a ready and waiting operating room, can bypass the ED completely and move toward the OR. Closed-loop communications with the ED and OR are critical to make this work. Our philosophy was that we would only stop in the emergency department if the patient's airway was immediately compromised. Even in a hypotensive patient, if they had a patent airway, we could initiate their operation quicker by bypassing the emergency department and going directly to the operating room. There were several excellent outcomes after this policy was implemented that proved its worth.

The philosophy of initial response and activation should revolve around early and rapid gathering of all potential necessary resources. To do this logically, you must identify those conditions that require rapid intervention and the presence of specialized personnel. If you extend the criteria beyond this you will begin to overtriage and create problems in your system.

Therefore the most obvious criteria are gunshots to the neck, abdomen, and chest; hypotensive patients; and those patients with obvious respiratory distress. The inclusion of low GCS patients in activation criteria is controversial. Though low GCS patients are part of the highest level activation criteria propagated by the American college of surgeons committee on trauma, there is not necessarily evidence to support that a trauma attending is necessary for these patients. Yet we must obey regulatory criteria. Of the criteria that many centers believe lead to overtriage, this is the greatest culprit.

There are only a few mandatory responders to the highest level activation that do not respond to a second tier activation (the trauma attending); however, an audit of the people notified of a highest level activation will usually find that up to ten personnel are expected to respond immediately. While there are some large and spacious trauma bays, 11 people in a 15 × 15 foot space, including equipment, stretcher, x-ray device, computer terminals, and a portable computer workstations will always lead to overcrowding. While many trauma directors are adamant about avoiding crowding in the trauma bay I think it is more important to make sure that people know their roles and carry them out efficiently. If there are spectators that can learn something and not interfere with the flow of the resuscitation, they should be allowed to observe. Should they become a hindrance, they must leave immediately when asked.

The American College of Surgeons committee on trauma has six mandatory activation criteria [1]. These include GCS eight or less with a mechanism of trauma, gunshot wound to the chest or abdomen, respiratory distress or field intubation, blood being transfused to maintain vital signs, emergency physician discretion, and hypotension less than 90 mmHg.

Many centers will expand on these but if you wish to be verified by the American College of Surgeons you must have all six of these.

Once you've created your criterion it is vitally important to make sure that everybody involved knows about them. It is also vital that there be an auditing system to determine whether people are activating the criteria appropriately. This is one of the greatest areas for integration with EMS. The vast majority of trauma patients interact with EMS before they interact with the trauma center. The most effective way to decrease lag time between injury and activation is to allow EMS to activate your trauma system. In our area we have printed out our first and second line activation criteria and asked it to be placed in all our regional ambulances. We've also empowered our advanced life support providers to call alpha and beta alerts (our top two levels of activation) independently and made it clear that we expect their wish to activate is respected. However this took a great deal of time (20 years) to convince emergency department faculty to trust the EMS providers' judgment regarding trauma team activation.

Psychologically one of the most difficult parts of the trauma surgeon/emergency physician relationship is convincing the emergency physicians that not only do you want to be called but you want to be called more than you're actually needed. As I said before, many emergency department personnel feel that the trauma team brings disruption to the emergency department. The background for this feeling should be investigated because they should not feel that way. Although I realize that the activation of the trauma team brings a large number of people into a room in the emergency department, we should provide sufficient value to make the department feel this is beneficial for all concerned. We should create this value by taking care of the patient in a thoroughly organized manner, and getting them through their diagnostic process quicker than if we had not been called. In our facility we audited this closely and over years we're able to demonstrate to the emergency department that when we were activated, the time that the patient spent the emergency department and the time that the patient occupied their personnel were decreased significantly. Once we were able to demonstrate this with actual data, we were able to convince them to call us when appropriate. However it is likely that in every center where a trauma medical director is trying to encourage trauma activation, they will have to go through some sort of learning interval where they will need to convince emergency department that they bring something useful to the game.

The best way to convince the ED you provide value is to:

- Have an organized trauma team response. This includes a briefing prior to arrival if possible with assignment of roles. All necessary equipment should be on hand and ready to be used.
- Integrate the ED team into the trauma team seamlessly by assigning roles and positions.
- Decide beforehand who will be doing what during the resuscitation to avoid conflict during patient care.
- Always put the patient first and not individual egos.
- Move efficiently through the process and move out of the ED as rapidly as safely possible (try not to return to the ED after moving to CT scan).
- An efficient system should have identified the likely destination of the patient after the secondary survey, chest x-ray, and focused abdominal sonography for trauma (FAST), and the hospital bed assignment should have been requested and should be ready by the time the advanced radiology tests are done.
- Handle conflict quietly and professionally.
- Control your residents to insure there is a solid chain of command, and not a diffusion of authority.
- Control your team to insure everyone understands the strategic plan (what you need to do in the next hour) and the tactical plan (what you need to do in the next 5 minutes).
- The team leader should never carry out tactical tasks (chest tubes, central lines) unless there is no other choice. By delving into the tactical, the team leader loses situational awareness.

Communications

While hospital care has almost completely ignored the advances in telecommunications in the past century, they are finally beginning to notice that the world has changed around them. Amazingly, we still use the same text paging systems in many healthcare systems that were used in 1970. There are centers that have experimented with a variety of modern techniques (direct connect phones, radios, Vocera, limited range secure phones) even the most advanced is probably 10 years behind the cutting edge (imagine using a 10-year-old iPhone for life-threatening situations or a 20-year-old cell phone).

This is important because we have found in our patient safety investigations that lapses in communication are the most common cause of reversible error in adverse events. The concept of a broadcast, horizontal, secure communication system in hospital medicine is almost unheard of, while it is used every day in the military and fire and police departments in the smallest town in the USA and throughout most of the industrialized world. Despite this, simple closed-loop real-time communications are not available in many hospitals.

There are good reasons why broadcast and closed-loop communication are used. First, they provide good situational awareness of all personnel involved in an incident. Second, in the event of a critical emergency, all that is needed is a press of a button to get help. It does not require calling an operator, looking up a pager number, creating a text message, etc. It also is closed loop, meaning that when you call for help, all the receiver needs to do is press a switch and say "I'm on my way, 2 minutes."

In my own setting, I have spent years and funds trying to implement an effective, efficient, reliable communication system. After several incidents where situational awareness and horizontal communications were missing, I undertook the study of our communication systems to see what could be done. Working with several system engineers, our conclusion was that a trunked, secure, radio system was the best solution. Our dream was that a small handheld device could be used to: announce trauma activations, insure clinician response, provide clinical updates, inform the ICU and OR of critical patients that needed their resources, coordinate care, and improve situational awareness in multiple patient incidents. In fact, even after short trial periods, our surveys found that the new system ameliorated all these issues.

But, as in many innovations, without constant prodding the radios were not worn or used. One chief resident simply said he didn't like it. When asked if he had tried it, he said no. So even after careful analysis, extensive product research, pilot periods, technological enhancement and coverage improvements, standard operating procedures, and instructional videos along with constant positive reinforcement, the project failed. So even a bad but familiar system will often persist when a newer better system exists if the new system requires adaptation. Trauma medical directors need to be aware of this fact when trying to implement change across a system.

Transfer Between Emergency Departments

Communication of the trauma patient's arrival through the emergency department is key to a successful outcome and organized trauma response. What can be frustrating for trauma directors is the reluctance of the emergency department to have a programmed, activation system due to the reasons I have already discussed. In many of the trauma centers that I've evaluated as well as my own certain emergency physicians are reluctant to allow prehospital providers to recommend a trauma activation on their own and reluctant to allow the people taking the prehospital information to activate an alert without having an ED attending in the loop.

There are some valid reasons for this, the first being that the emergency department attending must maintain situational awareness of everything going on in their department. Thus they feel that if prehospital providers or nurses/medical communications personnel are allowed to activate the trauma response on their own, then a situation may ensue where a critical trauma patient is arriving in the emergency department and they are not aware. However this is easily remedied, through an automatic communication with the emergency medicine attending, through direct connect phones, or through radio. In addition if the trauma response is well organized the emergency medicine attending should not require a great deal of warning for the arrival of the trauma patient. There should be a room set aside for these patients along with equipment, nurses and technicians. When we have done root cause analyses of suboptimal resuscitations and adverse outcomes in trauma patients in the ED, you often find that the root cause is delayed activation and delayed arrival of the team. As a trauma team leader, I have often found that if we arrive minutes after the patient has arrived in the emergency department, we feel like we are already behind the pace of events and are constantly catching up. When this occurs you don't have time for a briefing, assigning roles, or outlining a plan for a complex patient. It often requires a handoff between the emergency medicine team and the trauma team, which takes some time, and may often result in repeating certain aspects of the primary and secondary survey for the new team. The bottom line is, it is always better if the trauma team is in the emergency department before or at the arrival of the patient and arriving after the fact even as little as three or 4 minutes usually damages the efficiency of the process.

Trauma center verification criteria requires that there need to be a programmed communication process where either a medical communications person takes the information from prehospital and provides this to the EM attending or charge nurse. Those two personnel can then approve the activation of the alert and the alert ensues. As part of the PI process, it is often useful to look at the amount of warning that the trauma team gets for trauma activations either in individual cases that fall outside recommended parameters or in aggregate. This delay and lack of notification in a timely manner can be measured and can be improved.

As an example of why this system is so important, there are EMS systems where the prehospital personnel do not communicate directly with the emergency department. In a large city in the USA, EMS providers do not have radio communication with the emergency department and communicate critical patient information through a dispatcher who uses a landline. As you can imagine this is a suboptimal process for several reasons. First there may be minute by minute urgent updates that the incoming EMS unit must communicate to the trauma team, such as loss of airway, severe hypotension, or arterial bleeding. All of which may present themselves in the last few minutes of transport. In addition this process does not allow the emergency medicine staff to ask any questions of the incoming EMS unit simply because this would need to be relayed through the dispatcher and it is often discouraged.

Though this is an unusual system, it can be difficult to prove scientifically that this system causes adverse outcomes. As in many performance improvement projects the superiority of an optimal efficient process can often be difficult to demonstrate. Does this mean that if you cannot demonstrate the superiority of one process over another that we should allow complete variability and improvisation? My answer is no. Performance improvement and creation of optimal systems will always depend in some way on examination of steps in the process and optimization. If we were to spend all of our time collecting data on every process in the trauma center, we would have time to do nothing else. Sometimes you do need to look at what process is being used across many other centers effectively and demand that process be replicated unless there are extremely valid reasons why it should not be used.

Next is the communication with the trauma team. The most common method of this is pager communications. It is vital that these pager communications be set up as a group because there are usually at least eight to nine pagers that must be activated and activating each pager individually will usually take several minutes and waste a great deal of time. Almost every paging system allows the creation of paging groups that can send out all these pages with the same message at the same time. Other possibilities are direct connect phones and radio communication. Direct connect phones were thought to be the salvation of urgent hospital communications when they first came out; however, for several years there was no phone provider that would provide support for direct connect phones. Now there is one and we are seeing direct connect phones being used more often in trauma.

As far as radio communications using secure, trunked, transmission, is still very rare. The advantages of radio communication are similar to those of direct connect phones in that they provide a horizontal broadcast transmission capability all members of the team can receive the information at the same time without calling individuals. As I said previously, in my own center, we attempted to implement this and even after a year and a half are still having difficulty getting people who are not used to using radios to use them regularly.

The next topic is what should be communicated. I've seen wide variability in this from almost complete patient reports to simply "Trauma Alert." Since the team should be ready for anything a great deal of information is not required. But a last set of vital signs mechanism and the status of the airway and GCS are good minimum components of the report. This is also another reason why some emergency medicine attendings do not want EMS activation, because they feel the EMS providers would simply say trauma alert and will not provide any further information. However if you've been in this business for a while, you know that pre-hospital information can be inaccurate. In any trauma center, the trauma team should be prepared for what comes through the door as long as a team is assembled briefed and ready. In our own center, we provide a level of activation dependent on mechanism, last set of vital signs, GCS, and ETA. For a highest level activation, we want closed-loop communications with MEDCOM (our prehospital communications personnel) to ensure that the trauma attending is aware that an activation is on the way. We have also tried several other enhancements to this process. First emails are sent out to the trauma attending and trauma team whenever helicopters are dispatched for a trauma patient. This is of some utility, in that if the team is busy with other duties, and they know that helicopters are going to the scene or another hospital with the trauma patient, they can begin to organize tasks in such a way to ensure that they are free when the patient arrives. In addition for each activation, and we have three levels of activation (alpha, beta, and gamma) and an email is sent to the trauma attendings for each activation. We felt that a beep for all attendings, even those not on call would be a bit much, but all the attendings found the email is useful, even at night, to keep track of what is going on and as the backup attending to know what your services may be needed. Situational awareness is good, and increasing the situational awareness of the trauma staff is a positive.

Updating Trauma Center with New Patient Information

As I said before, the team should be ready for anything that comes through the door, but it is essential that certain changes in condition be communicated to the team as they happen. First, a change in airway and respiratory status must be communicated, while the airway resources should be present for a highest level activation, knowing that a patient has lost their airway in transit, or that the patient is now having severe respiratory distress, and preparation for immediate intubation, cricothyroidotomy, or thoracostomy tube placement can be enhanced with up-to-date information.

I have probably run close to 1000 EMS calls in the back of an ambulance, so I am aware of the extreme multitasking that goes on and that the trauma center cannot be unreasonable in asking for up-to-date information. Technology can address this issue. EMS systems have moved to headsets with simple Push to talk capabilities for the lead medic, so they can communicate with the hospital easily, without picking up a handset, or dialing an access code. Simple, 3–5 word updates are all that is needed in these situations, and the hospital should resist asking for more information when it is clear the medics are task saturated.

Assembly and Briefing

While at the beginning of my career, I was not a big fan of microscopically set procedures for trauma resuscitations, I am now convinced that time-outs and briefings improve efficiency, communication, and outcomes. In order to have a briefing, you need the team to be assembled (another reason why short notice or activation after the patient arrives are so suboptimal).

The briefing has several essential components: introductions and role (*OK, everyone, listen up; I'm Dr. Young; I'm the team leader, and all orders will come from me. Next...*). Go around the bed and have everyone introduce themselves and state their role.

Here is a typical briefing script:

- *Team leader:* "I am Dr. Smith, and I'll be the team leader; all orders should come through me. If someone attempts to give an order, ask me whether to do it or not. This is Dr. Young, he is the surgery attending and is in overall command, and this is Dr. Jones, the emergency medicine attending who will be working with us. Now, everyone introduce themselves and their role."
- *Primary nurse:* "I'm John Smith and I'll be the primary nurse."
- *Airway lead:* "I'm Dr. West and I'll be handling the airway and the head and neck exam."
- *Primary survey:* "I'm Bill North, I'm a medical student, and I'm doing the primary and secondary surveys."
- *Respiratory therapy:* "I'm Linda from respiratory therapy."
- *Procedure lead:* "I'm Dr. South and I'll be handling the FAST exam and procedures."

- *Recording nurse:* "I'm Julie and I'm the recording nurse."
- *Radiology tech:* "I'm Lisa from radiology."
- *Team leader:* "Great, so what we know is this is an elderly gentleman who suffered a ground level fall and was found unconscious; he was intubated by EMS at the scene; his blood pressure is 80/60, and pulse is 70; ETA is 5 minutes. Airway: make sure the tube is in the right place and the patient has good breath sounds and call out confirmation. Bill, call out the primary survey loudly so everyone can hear. If the patient's initial BP on our monitor is less than 90 we will initiate blood transfusion, is the blood in the room?"
- *Primary nurse:* "Yes the cooler is right behind me and the rapid infuser is ready to go."
- *Team leader:* "OK everyone, let's keep the noise level down, only speak out when you need to or unless you have an assignment and let's remember to call back any order that is was received and who is carrying it out. If things go badly either I or Dr. Young will be calling out commands and we are the only ones you should be listening to for orders. Let's go!"

Reference

1. Committee on Trauma, American College of Surgeons. Resource for optimal care of the injured patient, 2014. https://www.facs.org/-/media/files/quality-programs/trauma/vrc-resources/resources-for-optimal care.ashx?la–cn.

Chapter 6
First 5 Minutes

Handoff with EMS

We have done a lot of different things with the EMS handoff and have a current system that we think works well. First, some of the problems with the handoff must be recognized:

- The team is usually anxious to get their hands on the patient and ignores the EMS provider.
- The EMS provider doesn't know how to give an efficient, complete handoff.
- The team leader and the EMS provider have a "sidebar" handoff, and the entire team does not hear it.
- And most importantly, critical information is not transferred.

We examined the problem and came to the conclusion that if the transfer to the hospital bed is made before the handoff, the momentum is to move forward with the various tasks, and the handoff does not take place effectively. Thus, taking the time to have the handoff occur while the patient is still on the EMS gurney focuses everyone's attention and provides a pause. For those of you who may object to this pause, remember it only takes about 60 seconds, and there are very few

© Springer Nature Switzerland AG 2020 69
J. S. Young, *Trauma Centers*,
https://doi.org/10.1007/978-3-030-34607-2_6

patients where that minute is significant. However, our procedure is for the team leader to ask the lead medic when they walk in the room "is the airway and the patient stable?" If the medic says "no" then the patient is immediately transferred over, and the handoff occurs in the traditional fashion with the EMS provider trying to talk over the team doing tasks. We have found that this is necessary in less than one in ten cases.

So our process is:

- EMS provider immediately indicates to team if ABC's are not under control, and in that case, the patient is immediately transferred over, and care is initiated with the provider giving a handoff to the crowd as best they can.
- If ABC's are stable, everyone pauses and the EMS provider gives the report including:
- Age, sex
- Mechanism

  - With important details (death in passenger compartment, ejection, etc.)

- Initial ABCs and vital signs
- Apparent injuries
- Medical history or allergies (last meal? Who cares, you treat everyone like they have a full stomach)
- Final set of vital signs and meds given en route
- Questions?

Patient is transferred to ED stretcher with careful disconnection and movement of lines and monitors. We do not remove the EMS monitor until our monitors are in place.

Primary Survey, FAST, and CXR

We have similarly made many evolutional changes in the primary survey over the decades. In ATLS, you are taught that the primary survey is the sole responsibility of the lead clinician; however, in real life it is a shared responsibility. As it is in ATLS, airway, breathing, and circulation are the key factors in preventing early death in injured patients. Thus you need to make certain a trustworthy person is evaluating these aspects and, if not trustworthy, at least has someone "at the elbow" confirming the data.

Once the patient is on the ED stretcher, several processes should occur simultaneously. In actuality, even if you have more personnel, it doesn't help. There is only so much room around the stretcher and a limit to the number of things that can be going on without creating chaos.

Our process is that the person at the head of the bed calls out the primary survey:

- "Airway intact"
- "Breath sounds equal bilaterally"
- "Good carotid pulses"
- "Pupils equal and reactive"

Of course, you will immediately act on any critical problems in the primary survey immediately. I'll enumerate some of my strategies and hints for each.

Airway

Trauma surgeons and EM physicians (and anesthesiologists) often differ on indications for intubation in the acute trauma patient. I have always preferred the patient to arrive intubated by the aeromedical or ground crew, as long as the tube is in the trachea.

Our philosophy is to put safety first, even if it is *possible* that the patient could persist without intubation in radiology, we would rather be certain that the patient is OK before leaving the bay. The old maxim "death begins in radiology" can be obviated by having an intubated and lined up patient (especially with an arterial line). So we intubate patients:

- In shock
- With significant facial injuries that are causing any airway compromise
- Unable to follow commands

We will also intubate if:

- The patient is a danger to themselves by not allowing us to diagnose and treat injuries, if they are not lucid.
- The patient is having significant vomiting and any evidence of aspiration.
- If we are unable to provide lifesaving treatment due to extreme pain. Meaning that painful procedures are necessary (such as joint relocations), and we are too concerned about the patient's hemodynamic status to prescribe sufficient pain control and sedation.
- Burn patients with significant intraoral burns or significant stridor and/or voice change.
- Patient with cervical spine injuries and no evidence of chest wall movement with breathing.

Of course, there are many other possible reasons, but these are the highlights.

The process of intubation can be complex and dangerous. Some patients will crash on induction due to hypovolemia, vomit, and rapidly desaturate. Also, the routine practice of having novice EM and anesthesia residents taking the first good look at the cords, and then transitioning the patient to a high tension, high anxiety intubation at the hands of the senior resident or attending is unfortunately commonplace.

It goes without saying that you need a recent blood pressure (hopefully accurate), reliable pulse oximetry readings, a solid IV, suction, bougie, at least two ET tube sizes, and a working laryngoscope. The discussion of intubation aids such as a GlideScope device are beyond the scope of this work, but I think the most reliable intubation technique is a clinician with experience in airway control, good relaxation, good equipment, and the focus of everyone in the room to augment the evolution.

Difficult Airway/Intubation Failure

Airway loss/massive aspiration and brain damage or death are major causes of lawsuits in trauma, not to mention the devastating effect on patients and families. I think one of the major problems with difficult airways is that there are not always clear cut signs for moving to the next step in the algorithm. For instance, when a patient begins to desaturate during an intubation attempt, at what point do you stop and bag the patient? While this may seem straightforward (bag before the patient becomes bradycardic and suffers cardiac arrest), in practice it can be difficult especially with someone at the head who you know to be competent. If the intubating clinician is a novice, you are more likely to move to the next step earlier.

Since the first attempt at the airway is often the best chance, you want that person to be able to adjust and suction adequately to get a good view. What if they have suctioned, changed their blade position and are about to advance, when the saturations drop to 60%? Do you immediately order them to stop and bag, when you know there is a possibility that getting the airway on this attempt may be the best shot? What if I tell them to bag mask ventilate, and they say "I got it, just give me 2 seconds"? If its someone you trust, you will give them that time, if it is someone inexperienced you will not. But what if even the inexperienced person finally has the view they need, and the tube properly positioned? Do you stop and start over, knowing the risk of aspiration has increased, and knowing another episode of hypoxia is likely?

Many of these questions are rhetorical. Of course, you stop if the saturations are dropping rapidly, but it can be a very difficult decision, and for the team leader, you only have one piece of information (the oxygen saturations) while the proceduralist has more information (the view, amount of secretions, good angle, etc.). My advice is beforehand to have a plan. For instance, "Jane, if the sats drop to 80%, we're bagging, OK?" and then you hold each other to it. If the sats are 79% and Jane says she needs another few seconds, then say "you have 5 seconds and we're bagging"; don't let it drag on. There will be times when you will need to use command voice to stop someone from continuing to flail and start using a bag mask to bring the patient's saturations up.

Surgical Options

I have done many surgical airways in the ED and field, and it is often striking that after flailing with orotracheal intubation for minutes, a competent surgeon can get a surgical airway in 5 seconds. However, the risk of bleeding is significant, damage to the larynx is higher than with an orotracheal intubation, and you are making a new wound.

So what is the moral of the story? Protect the patient from harm. My wife is an excellent obstetrician, and she has often said no family will ever get mad at you for giving them a healthy baby, even if it takes a cesarean section, whereas they are not going to thank you for avoiding a C-section if you give them a severely damaged child.

Since a competent general surgeon should be able to get a cricothyroidotomy in place for virtually any patient, quickly, then no patient should die with a general surgeon at the bedside from the inability to get the airway. Now this doesn't mean that you go to the surgical option regularly, but it means that your team should set limits (or at least set limits in your own mind) as to when you are going to abandon intubation and proceed to a surgical airway.

Another lifesaving option that is used far more often in prehospital care is supraglottic airways (laryngeal mask airways, King and esophageal airways). In the hospital, it is often considered beneath an EM physician or anesthesiologist to use such a rescue airway, but I have seen them save lives in numerous situations. Whether to use an LMA or King airway or do a surgical airway is up to the individual. If you are unable to intubate due to vomit, bleeding, etc., then the surgical airway is probably best. If visualization and anatomy are the issue, then an LMA or King may suffice. It has taken a long time for me to convince my team that a King airway that is in place and functioning is safe for intrahospital transport. If the EMS crew almost lost the patient and saved them with a King or LMA, it makes little sense to me to put the patient through that 20 minutes later if their saturations and end tidal (or ABG) are fine. Get the patient through their initial workup and then change out the tube when things have stabilized.

Breathing

Next we come to breathing. In many cases this is handled by examining the chest, looking at the pulse oximetry tracing and the chest x-ray, but I would be remiss if I didn't discuss some of the critical issues in the primary survey breathing evaluation.

First, when the patient rolls in, the team leader (and really everyone) should be paying attention to the patient's breathing pattern. If the patient is being bag mask ventilated, then it's time to draw up the intubation drugs (usually etomidate and succinylcholine), make certain your lines are working, and get the patient intubated. It is highly unlikely you will be able to avoid intubation in a trauma patient who arrived with the ventilations assisted, unless they are fighting with the medic to "get the darn mask out of my face I'm trying to tell you I'm fine." And even in some of those cases, an intubation may be needed, but you have more time to evaluate and make the decision.

The examination of the chest is under- and overrated. In most EDs during a resuscitation, making fine discrimination between types of breath sounds is futile. However the presence of absence of breath sounds is determinable in most cases. Remember that in patients with large chests, or subcutaneous air, it can be difficult for sounds to be transduced (though the presence of subcutaneous air should tip you off that something untoward is going on).

There are often difficult decisions to make regarding the breathing portion of the first 5 minutes. For instance, the following adaptations of true cases are illustrative:

1. *A 50-year-old man is brought in after an MVC. He is awake but confused and moves all extremities. He is clearly in respiratory distress. The decision is made to intubate the patient and this is extremely complex, requiring a cricothyroidotomy. After the crich is confirmed to be in place with breath sounds and end tidal CO_2, we are unable to get the patients saturations above 80%. Breath sounds are present bilaterally and a stat CXR reveals the airway to be in good position, with abnormal lung fields bilaterally, but no evidence of collapse or massive fluid in either thorax. Despite*

*bag masking and suctioning, the saturations remain below
80%, BP is stable for the time being. While the possibility of
a pulmonary embolus is entertained, there is no history of
clotting disorders and DVTs, and EKG is grossly normal.
Chest tubes are placed bilaterally due to the dire situation.
There is no air or significant fluid from either thorax. An
ICU ventilator and oscillating ventilator are called down to
ED emergently to attempt more advanced ventilator management, the patient was deemed far too unstable to move to
ICU or CT scan. Simultaneously, cardiothoracic surgery is
contacted for the possibility of ECMO. However during the
ensuing minutes, the patient suffers a cardiac arrest and can-
not be resuscitated.*

2. *A 70-year-old man on Coumadin falls downstairs. He is
GCS 15 and hemodynamically stable in the ED. There is
bruising of the left chest and CXR reveals a moderate hemo-
thorax on the left without obvious pneumothorax. There are
no other fractures and FAST is negative. The patient is
breathing comfortably, and the decision is made to go to CT
to determine whether this finding on CXR is mostly fluid or
pulmonary contusion. While in CT the patient becomes
acutely hypotensive. The patient is pulled from CT and a left
chest tube is placed in the CT scanner. There is return of
800 cc of blood and within minutes the patient becomes
moribund. The patient is intubated, the massive transfusion
protocol is activated, and patient returned to ED. The patient
arrests and a left thoracotomy is performed. There is a massive contusion of the lower left lobe with what appears to be
intercostal bleeding and hemorrhage into the lung. Despite
efforts, the patient does not survive.*

Both these cases demonstrate that the breathing portion
of the algorithm can require urgent and hyper-urgent
decision-making and action and that in certain circumstances,
you may be acting prophylactically to prevent later
deterioration.

After the airway is confirmed, auscultation of both lung
fields and an external exam should be performed and called
out to the team. Bruising, deformity, flail segments, crepitus

and subcutaneous emphysema are all significant findings. For penetrating trauma, the entire thorax (including axilla and lower neck) should be scrupulously examined, and findings should be communicated to the team leader.

The breathing examination must always be done while being aware of the patient's clinical respiratory status. A patient without external signs of injury, who is gasping for air and is in extremis, may represent a patient with emphysema who has ruptured a bleb and is developing a tension pneumothorax. On the other hand, a patient with massive bruising who is breathing comfortably may require little or no intervention.

As I may have said previously, fear of devastating deterioration and complications can be an effective driver of treatment and protocol development in trauma care. With thoracic injuries, though the risk of life-threatening hemorrhage is low in the hospital setting, the risk of respiratory deterioration is significant. This can occur in the ED, or later that day, or a few days later. Thus, much of the treatment for breathing problems (which include thoracic injuries) is often preventative and involves intervening before physiology is significantly affected.

Getting back on track for the first 5 minutes, patients with an abnormal physical examination of the chest, who have oxygen saturations greater than 90% on room air (though patients who are 90% on 100% supplemental oxygen may be heading rapidly toward deterioration), can certainly wait for a chest x-ray before any interventions. This is just on the breathing side, if the patient has those saturations but is unconscious, or has an obstructing airway, that needs to be addressed immediately.

Other than intubation, interventions for breathing issues in the primary survey really only involve supplemental oxygen or a chest tube/dart. I am not a believer in darts (thoracic needle decompression) in the hospital setting. Any ED doc or surgeon (resident) should be able to wipe off the fifth intercostal space with betadine, make a 1 cm incision, and break into the pleural space with a Kelly clamp. If you say that it is medieval to do that without taking time to properly anesthetize the patient, I would say that if the patient is awake and cognizant enough to worry about that, then you don't need a needle decompression or hyper-urgent drainage, and you can take the proper time to prep, drape, and anesthetize the patient and put in a chest tube properly. This is only for the crashing patient with critically low oxygen saturations and severe respiratory distress where your physical exam or FAST leads you to believe you have a tension pneumothorax.

Chest Tubes

Chest tubes (thoracostomy tubes) have been placed for over 100 years. Yet they are one of the most difficult bedside procedures in trauma. I have seen chest tubes placed entirely outside of the thoracic cage (and not picked up for days), placed through one chest into the other, lacerate the heart, lacerate intercostal arteries (multiple times), increase bleeding, hit the thoracic duct, hit the azygos vein, etc. This is outside of the fact that it can be an extremely painful procedure.

Even more than central lines, I feel chest tube placement should be supervised by someone who has placed at least a dozen. From that experience, someone has probably seen enough variations to realize when things are getting dicey. I will not go into all the vagaries of placement here, but will touch on a few key points.

Always be aware of where you are on the chest: I have seen a half dozen chest tubes placed in the abdomen and have been an expert witness in cases where a spleen and a liver were lacerated leading to catastrophe. It is always better to place the tube too high rather than too low. If you place it too high, you may injure something high in the chest, but that is still better than inserting a chest tube through the diaphragm and abdominal organs. An even better idea is to put it in the right place.

Some of my maxims:

1. Never try to direct an unguided chest tube to a specific collection. If you need a guided chest tube, do it with ultrasound or CT guidance. The ability to guide a chest tube by just bending it and hoping almost always leads to a kinked tube, or one that has now gone through the lung. I tell residents "Fifth intercostal space between mid- and anterior axillary line every time." Don't go low to get an inferior collection, you'll fail.

2. Always sweep the inside of the chest with your finger before placement. You need to make certain you have a clear space to place the tube, another method to avoid sticking it through the lung.

3. Direct tube superiorly and posteriorly every time. Don't aim for a collection. A properly placed dependent tube will work 90% of time. If it doesn't, you need guided drainage.

4. Use the whole syringe of Lidocaine. I think it's very hard to make it painless, but it shouldn't be torture. Also, the local anesthetic should be supplemented with intravenous pain medication either fentanyl or ketamine.

5. Cut the end of tube across before hooking into the drainage tube, don't invert or let drainage apparatus lie on side (common when switching to OR table). Tape connections. Suture tube with TWO separate sutures 180° apart. Take tube securely to chest. Obtain an immediate post-procedure CXR and examine it carefully.

Chapter 7
Second Diagnostic Phase: First 30 Minutes

Execution

The execution of the time after the first 5 minutes of ABCs and resuscitation can be critical. This is the time where you are often deciding whether to take the patient to the operating room, where you are considering skipping certain routine diagnostic tests due to the condition of the patient, and where consultants will often be pushing the trauma team in different directions. This is also the time where the patient's family has arrived, and where you are dealing with loved ones who have just found out their family member is in critical condition when they were eating breakfast with them just a few hours earlier.

Keys to execution in the first 30 minutes are:

- Set a plan for this time period and insure that everyone knows what that plan is.

  - *"Ok everyone, listen up, we have the airway secured, we have a good chest x-ray, we have our lines and the BP seems stable. We're going to CT for pan scan and barring any new findings the patient is going to the SICU. Lets bring the trauma blood with us. Let ortho know we're going to the scanner and if they want they can do a quick exam there"*

© Springer Nature Switzerland AG 2020   81
J. S. Young, *Trauma Centers*,
https://doi.org/10.1007/978-3-030-34607-2_7

- Prepare for the worst.

  - Insure you are bringing personnel, medications, and equipment to intervene should something dire occur
  - Two large IVs
  - Sedatives
  - Fluids
  - Blood (and rapid infuser if quasi-stable)
  - Nurses
  - Respiratory therapy
  - Good MD help

    - Naturally I am referring to the critical trauma patient here, not the extremely stable, minimally injured patient undergoing a routine workup

- Treat potentially life-threatening injuries prior to transport to radiology.

  - Pneumothoraces seen on CXR
  - Significant hemothoraces
  - External bleeding dripping off bed or soaking sheets or dressings

- If the patient is not intubated, insure you can safely sedate the patient, and if possible, allow time for orthopedics to place fracture in rough alignment and splint (if unstable, skip this, but you need limbs in position such that patient can be placed in CT).
- Be ready for contingencies.

  - Respiratory distress
  - Hypotension

Consults and Delays

Consultants have a tendency to confuse things since they are responsible for a single system and not the entire patient. Often when you are looking for a straightforward answer from neurosurgery or orthopedics, you will get equivocation. This can be a real problem when you are juggling multiple life-threatening priorities, and you need to make a plan.

For instance, the classic situation is the patient who presents GCS 3, intubated, no movement for EMS, scattered respiratory effort, whose head CT comes off and shows questionable uncal herniation and a very tight brain, without a SDH (subdural hematoma) or EDH (epidural hematoma) that could be operated on. The next scan that comes off shows an abdomen with significant intraperitoneal fluid and a shattered spleen. Coincident with this, the patient's BP drops into the 80s. Neurosurgery says "I think this is a fatal head injury, but I can't say for sure," and you need to decide whether to run someone up to the OR for a laparotomy who may have an unrecoverable brain injury. But you can't let the patient bleed to death without definitive conclusions from neurosurgery. As many experienced trauma surgeons know, sometimes you do need to open these patients and stop their bleeding even though their chance of neurologic recovery is nearly zero.

Another situation is orthopedics wishing to reduce a hip or shoulder before moving the patient to the scanner. Making this worse, is consciously sedating a patient with unknown abdominal and head injuries. Do you leave the hip displaced? Do you rapidly intubate the patient to allow the hip to be reduced quickly and to protect the airway in a patient that is yet undiagnosed? Do you risk deep conscious sedation in a patient that has not yet had a head CT?

If the patient's limbs are so badly angulated that you can't fit the patient in the scanner, then ortho needs to be given the time to place betadine soaked gauzes on the open fractures and straighten the limb and apply a splint. Any more than that is wasting time and creating inertia. If the patient is awake and their limbs need to be straightened, you can try ketamine or fentanyl/Versed for conscious sedation, but as I said previously, doing this in a patient where intracavitary bleeding has not been ruled out is very dangerous. Usually in those cases we perform rapid sequence intubation (RSI) and intubate the patient for safety.

The bottom line to prevent problems in these situations is someone in command who has good situational awareness, and who can take an honest look at the competing priorities and competently put them in order. This is where I often see non-trauma surgeons and EM physicians fall short. You need the experience to be able to put things in perspective and tell senior consultants "no you're going to have to wait until we finish the workup." It is difficult to properly order these priorities without the experience of seeing many multiple trauma patients through their entire hospital course.

A simple way to look at this dilemma is to imagine the worst condition you may find is actually present (grade V splenic laceration with extravasation, for instance). Would you really want to try to justify why you wasted 30 minutes in the trauma bay suturing a scalp laceration when someone is bleeding into their belly? While you might say that's unlikely, then why are you obtaining the test if you believe there is no chance it will find something significant?

There are only a few consultant issues of overriding, or high priority:

- An ENT issue related to airway and tracheal injury needs to be dealt with in the bay. Again, you do not want to be in radiology with a tracheal fracture closing off the airway or a neck hematoma expanding. A simple way to settle this priority is intubation, and sometimes that is the quickest and simplest process. Prophylactic intubations are a real phenomenon and are often life preserving. In fact, I would argue many trauma bay intubations are prophylactic, to prevent deterioration, to allow sedation for pain, etc.
- The only overriding orthopedic issue is severe external bleeding. Remember life always comes before limb, so even if a limb is pulseless, that does not take priority of life-threatening bleeding or brain injury. But I have many anecdotes of patients where EMS placed large bulky gauze dressings around an open femur or tib/fib fracture and hidden 3–5 units of blood loss. These dressings MUST be taken down quickly (trauma shears) and redressed properly. You do not want to be able to follow your patient to CT by their trail of blood down the hallway. This is especially true of scalp wounds where the patient arrives with a huge gauze head wrap of bandages that when removed

end up weighing 5 pounds. Instruct your EMS people and ED people the key to stopping bleeding is the 4 Ps – pinpoint, prompt, precise, and pressure. We also use the Israeli combat dressing and QuikClot gauze to great effect. It is small and easy to apply, and I have seen it stop everything short of an arterial bleed.

- In that vein do not take someone to the scanner with an obvious arterial bleeder. Get a big stitch and stop it. Then after things calm down, take the dressing down, prep, anesthetize, drape, and properly wash out and repair the laceration. This is a stopgap measure to get you to the scanner.

Destination Plan

This is the point where a great deal of inertia can be avoided by assigning the patient's inpatient unit. By getting the process of obtaining an ICU bed going, you can avoid coming back to the ED from radiology. A good rule to practice by is that once a multi-trauma leaves the ED, they should not return.

Contingency Planning

The team leader and team members should always plot out contingencies before leaving the ED. What if the small pneumothorax leads to respiratory distress? What if the patient becomes hypotensive? What if the patient requires intubation?

In our system, the team and a pharmacist accompany the nurse and patient to radiology. In this way we can get access to medications rapidly. They usually travel with intubation and sedation medications. An airway box should be available at your destination.

Emergency blood usually accompanies highest level activations. This blood should not be returned to the blood bank until intracavitary bleeding is ruled out in a patient with any evidence of instability. I have seen many cases where a patient looked stable after a liter of saline, but who crashed in CT and the blood was now back in the blood bank delaying transfusion.

We believe that pneumothoraces and hemothoraces visible on chest x-ray should be drained in the trauma bay before going to CT. We have had adverse events where patients with small pneumothoraces became unstable in CT, and there was significant delay in bringing the patient back to the ED for a thoracostomy tube, or bringing the necessary equipment to CT. Put the tube in before you leave the bay. If you are going directly to the OR and the patient is oxygenating, and there is no evidence of tension physiology, it is often easier to place the tube in the OR once the patient is asleep.

The Hyper-Urgent Patient

A term our center and others have used is hyper-urgent, which attempts to differentiate the routine "emergent" patient which encompasses a wide range of clinical conditions (from ruptured appendix to leaking aneurysm), many of which can be treated in a 2–8 hour time frame, from those patients where 5–10 minutes mean the difference between life and death.

The hyper-urgent patient should be identified by prehospital report (*this is rescue 143, we have a 19-year-old male with a gunshot wound to the abdomen, he s somnolent and has a weak radial pulse, be there in 5 minutes*). This patient requires little if any time in the ED, since their life will be saved in the operating room. The only reason to stop in the ED for these patients is to secure an airway, if the airway is untenable. But if you are able to manage the airway non-invasively, it is safer to run the patient up to the OR and induce when you are prepped and ready to open the abdomen in case the patient crashes.

Hyper-urgent patients truly demonstrate the level of performance of the ED and OR phases of your trauma center. A center that cannot go directly to the OR with a patient like this is inadequate. A center that cannot bring this patient into a trauma bay, intubate, and roll them out of the bay in less than 10 minutes has problems. This is not the totality of a center's worth, but any hospital calling itself a trauma center must be able to handle these patients seamlessly.

The Multiple Priority Hyper-Urgent Patient

These patients separate the average solid trauma center from the exceptional center. Our motto is that we need to save everyone we should save and half the patients that can't be saved. To do that, you must be able to save these critically injured, multiple priority, and unstable patients regularly. Below are examples:

- The blunt trauma patient with a shattered pelvis, open extremity fracture, positive FAST, low GCS, and hypotension
- The blunt or penetrating trauma patient who has aspirated or suffered some other respiratory embarrassment and can't be ventilated or oxygenated
- The blunt patient with a blown pupil, major thoracic injuries, and a positive FAST
- The penetrating trauma patient with life-threatening injuries in multiple cavities (skull, chest, abdomen, pelvis)

The team leader/trauma surgeon who can effectively handle these patients not only has knowledge but must have experience, command presence, and the ability to make critical decisions quickly and confidently.

Communication and the Hyper-Urgent Patient

Communication is also an essential part of caring for these patients. Often critical information must be shared with the OR, blood bank, interventional radiology, and multiple consultants. Ingrained programmed processes are probably the best way to avoid communication failures. If people know the recommended sequence of events and know their roles, then it is less likely that they will make errors. However, good real-time tactical communications are as important in caring for the trauma patient as they are when commanding an accident or fire scene. Since physicians and nurses have little experience with tactical communications (radios) this form of communications in the hospital has lagged. Beeping or calling six separate individuals to get a patient set up for an emergency laparotomy is a recipe for delays and miscommunication.

The lack of closed loop communications is also a major issue. Paging systems and texts are open loop meaning that you do not KNOW that the recipient received and understood the message. In fire/EMS/Police communications, read-back of the message is mandatory and indicates to the sender that the message was received and understood. Hopefully we can integrate these types of communication into trauma care, but as someone who has tried to innovate in this area, it has been extremely painful and slow.

Open-loop communications in these situations can be deadly. For instance, the team leader says to the trauma bay "make sure we have 4 units of FFP in the OR." Our typical process is someone may say "OK," and the team leader never sees who acknowledged, and there is usually no loop closure that the task is done. In fire/EMS this communication would be:

- *Medic 1: "We need a second medic unit at this scene"*
- *911 Center: "Understood Medic 1 you need another medic unit at highway 64 mile marker 229?"*
- *Medic 1: "Affirmative"*
- *911 Center: "911 Direct"*

- *911 Center: "Medic 1?"*
- *Medic 1: "Medic 1"*
- *911 Center: "Medic 504 is en route, ETA 5 minutes"*
- *Medic 1: "Medic 1 understood"*

While this seems complex, it is second nature to fire/EMS and should become second nature to us. In actuality paging systems are probably the most dangerous communication system at this moment. Push to talk, secure messaging, secure cell phones, or radio communications are all superior.

Transition Phase: ED to ICU and Initial Critical Care – Second 30 Minutes to 2 Hours

We are now at the 30-minute mark. ABCs have been evaluated and treated, initial plain x-rays and labs are done and have been reviewed, and CT scans are coming up on the monitor. This is the point where in the urgent (not emergent or hyper-urgent) patient, the true treatment plan is constructed and implemented.

In the 30- to 120-minute period, many critical decisions will be made:

- Where is the family and have they been informed? What advance directives are in place?
- Can the patient go for orthopedic fixation or traction and splinting?
- Do they need lacerations repaired in ED or should it be done in the OR?
- Do they need ICP monitoring? How can we follow a neurologic examination safely?
- Can they wean to extubation in the next few hours, or do we need to mechanically ventilate for the time being?
- Do they need follow-up imaging, and is it safe to transport them for this imaging?
- What lab and radiology studies do we need in the short term? How will we change our plan based on these results?
- What consultant recommendations need to be discussed and how will we prioritize what needs to be done?

While there are infinite ways that people can be injured, after two decades of treating trauma patients on a daily basis, these are the major categories:

- Major head injuries
- Multiple orthopedic injuries

- Major chest
- Major abdomen
- Major spine
- Life-threatening multiple trauma (Big crunch)

This may seem simplistic, but for each patient, there needs to be first priorities and second and third priorities. Some things need to take precedence over others when deciding how to sequence your actions.

For instance, in the typical multiple trauma, there are usually chest injuries (rib fractures, hemo/pneumothorax), orthopedic injuries (most commonly femur, pelvis, or tibia), and head injury (small amounts of subdural or subarachnoid blood and alterations in consciousness). Thankfully in the hemodynamically and neurologically stable patient, rapid cross-sectional imaging through CT scanning of the head, neck, chest, abdomen, and pelvis allows you to rule out life-threatening issues in less than 30 minutes from arrival on many cases. This allows thoughtful prioritization of treatment.

Errors usually occur when data is inaccurate, or not properly analyzed. For instance, when FAST first came into use, the number of non-therapeutic laparotomies increased. This was due to the perception that a positive FAST in a stable patient represented active abdominal bleeding, when all it was showing was the presence of fluid. For decades before that, we were CT scanning abdomens and finding fluid and solid organ injury, over 90% of which could be managed non-operatively [1]. Logically, all positive FAST in a stable patient was telling us that there was fluid in their abdomen, and in the stable patient operative intervention is not usually necessary. Thus, a new data acquisition method was not being used logically.

So while you have hopefully ruled out issues that will immediately kill the patient, there are still significant problems in this phase that can cause the patient's demise, either that day or several days later.

Major Head Injuries

The vast majority of severe head injuries do not go immediately to the operating room for treatment. Most go to the ICU for ICP monitoring and medical management of ICP. In these cases, neurosurgery will always prefer that sedation be minimized so a neurologic exam can be followed. This is logical since if the patient can follow commands, their continued ability to follow commands bodes well for their cerebral function.

However, this is not always possible. Patients with multiple trauma often have painful injuries that require analgesia and sedation. Procedures need to be performed including major laceration repair, operative management of injuries, or pinning and traction on fractures if it is unsafe to go to OR. Thus, guaranteeing that the patient will always be examinable is often impossible. What always causes me great concern is that sedation will be required for a short period (let's say 90 minutes) for procedures with the expectation that it can be turned off for an exam. What happens not infrequently is that when the sedation is turned off, the exam has changed, and at this point you do not know if it is the result of residual sedation effect or an increasing mass lesion. You also don't know if the exam changed 5 minutes ago or 95 minutes ago. This is why traumatologists will often push the neurosurgeons to place ICP monitoring in these patients. The neurosurgeons rightly push back that the scientific evidence for ICP monitoring is weak, and it can cause problems of its own. In truth an ICP monitor may be looked back on in 30 years like a wooden club, but it's all we have.

If operative neurosurgical intervention is required in this time period, it of course must be allowed, and trauma needs to do everything we can to insure the patient gets through the operation safely. But even in the most unstable patient, emergent craniotomy must be allowed for a worsening neurologic injury. If the patient is unstable due to bleeding in the abdomen and chest, simultaneous procedures can be performed, though if you have no standard work for this process, it will not be smooth. Saving the body while allowing the brain to die does no one any good.

If there is a serious brain injury, but operative management is not immediately indicated, this is the time period where bad things can happen. This is the time where the patient is often getting follow-on studies (angiography, MRI, etc.) and procedures as detailed above. For a patient with a tight brain, this is often a time where the pCO_2 is poorly controlled, and where hypertonic saline treatment is not occurring. Also, pain may be poorly controlled as well as sedation. This is why it is vital in these types of critical patients to move them from the CT scanner to the SICU and NOT back to the ED. Getting the patient in the SICU where they can be under the treatment of critical care nurses and respiratory therapists experienced in treating severe brain injury is critical. Spending more time in the relatively uncontrolled environment of the ED should only be done when absolutely necessary.

Since many of our most seriously injured patients suffer head injuries, our program has spent a great deal of time and energy trying to decrease variability in neurotrauma care. The problem is the evidence to mandate any course of action is poor. We know hypoxia and hypotension are not good for the injured brain, but other than that the evidence supporting any drug, procedure, or intervention is poor. We do our best to avoid huge bumps in the road, which is why we practice early aggressive airway control, invasive arterial monitoring, and rapid neurosurgical consultation. Our current standard (as outline in our manual) is to use hypertonic saline to bring the serum sodium to >145, to maintain a pCO_2 of 33–36 mmHg, insure complete sedation or paralysis if necessary, elevate the head of the bed if possible, and avoid compression of the jugular veins. Any mass lesion undergoes a repeat head CT within 4 hours.

Multiple Orthopedic Injuries

Orthopedic injuries can be interesting to look at but are rarely life-threatening. Every trauma team leader has had to tell team members or spectators to put down their cell phone cameras taking pictures of the mangled and backward extremity and go back to the ABCs. A rapid evaluation for major hemorrhage should be done as part of D (disability) and E (exposure) in the ABCs. This is what tactical combat casualty care training refers to as getting the patient "trauma naked" and examining each extremity to insure there is no uncontrolled bleeding. This would be evidenced by pooling blood on the stretcher, spurting blood, etc. This needs to be acted upon rapidly especially if there's evidence of arterial hemorrhage. Many EDs prior to the BCON (bleeding control) course did not have adequate functional tourniquets available, leading to large bandages over arteries and a lot of blood on the floor. What's good for the field regarding arterial hemorrhage is good for the ED and a tourniquet should be placed immediately, and they should be readily available.

If a patient has a high-risk injury (GSW or stab wounds through area of vascular traverse, history of spurting hemorrhage, massive blood loss at the scene) and a tourniquet is in place, I am very wary of removing this device in the ED. First in a shocky, cold patient, the wound may not bleed initially but will bleed when the patient goes to the scanner or angiography with the tourniquet off. Then as the patient warms and their BP increases, bleeding begins again and can be massive. I believe in this modern Level I age, the patient should have vascular consultation, plain x-rays, and a trip to the OR or even better an OR hybrid room. Then an on-table angiogram can be performed with the leg prepped and draped, and the tourniquets can be removed with minimum continuing blood loss.

If there is no evidence of life-threatening hemorrhage but a variety of oozing wounds and new joints, move on. Do not spend time splinting or doing complex wound care until the "first 5 minutes" are done. Then after the primary, secondary surveys, FAST, and CXR are done and you know you have a stable patient, or a quasi-stable patient with a plan, you can move on to washing out and splinting fractures. But this should be done within 10 minutes. A trauma center that sees a lot of orthotrauma such as ours should have procedures in place for rapid splinting.

Orthopedic injuries are never a primary operative priority. They are a secondary priority after hemodynamic stability is attained, and intracranial, intrathoracic, and intra-abdominal life-threatening injuries are excluded. An exception to this are unstable pelvic fractures. Pelvic fractures are a subject of their own and can take their own chapter, but I will try to hit the high points.

Pelvic fractures usually bleed from arteries (in the back), veins (in the front), or both. Fractures where the pelvic volume is greatly increased (AC II or AC III), Malgaigne fractures, and fractures or conditions where the sacroiliac joints are "popped" are the most likely to cause life-threatening hemorrhage [2]. I believe if you handle things calmly and competently, your mortality rate from major pelvic fractures should be low. This includes:

- Large bore IV lines and immediate transfusion of blood for hypotension
- Stabilization of pelvis for anterior injuries using a commercially available stabilization device
- Careful FAST exam
- If quasi-stable and FAST negative – CT then angiography with binder in place
- If unstable and FAST negative – angiography with binder in place
- If unstable and FAST positive – OR, laparotomy, rapid pelvic stabilization by ortho, and then possible angiography depending on what you find in abdomen

There are centers practicing pelvic packing in these quasi- and unstable patients. This is not the standard nationally, and I have only seen it used in the minority of Level I centers I inspect, but it is something to consider and to keep track of in the literature [3].

Major Chest

Stable

Major chest injuries can be especially challenging, in that patients usually present either stable or gloriously unstable. For the stable patient, they usually have single or multiple rib fractures, pulmonary contusion, and/or hemothorax/pneumothorax. In 99% of these cases, in the first few hours, thoracostomy tube placement and assessment for need for ventilator support, and judicious pain control are the key maneuvers.

It is frequently difficult to predict which patients will survive without critical care and which will not. I've seen burly construction workers need mechanical ventilation with two rib fractures, and little old ladies smile at me with eight rib fractures. For many years we used the incentive spirometer as a simple test. If they could inhale a volume of greater than 1000 cc in the ED we put them on the floor. If it was between 500 and 1000, we put them in a stepdown unit. In both units, our respiratory therapists had a standard intensive therapy regimen for these patients. There are many maneuvers that are variably available to help such as rib blocks with long acting local anesthetics, and epidurals, but these are often not available in the first hour.

The Battle score is often used [4], and we implemented it in our institution in 2017. It seemed to place many patients in the ICU that we did not put there previously, but we have not yet validated its utility. We are currently analyzing these patients.

Pulmonary Contusion, Hemothorax, and Pneumothorax

Through some adverse events, we implemented the rule that hemothoraces and pneumothoraces seen clearly on the initial CXR in the trauma bay should be drained before the patient leaves the bay. We have had patients deteriorate while lying flat in CT with known hemo/pneumothoraces thus we created this rule. Obviously effusions and PTX that appear very small can go to CT without a chest tube.

Pulmonary contusion is also very common. A good rule of thumb is if you see what appears to be a contusion on AP (anterior-posterior) CXR, worry, if you only see it on CT, then you will probably have less trouble. Obviously pulmonary contusion, rib fractures, and blood in the chest in a patient with COPD or poor pulmonary reserves or CHF can turn a stable situation into an unstable one.

Major Abdomen

Outside of penetrating trauma, major combined abdominal injuries are not that common. In addition, rushing patients in the operating room for blunt abdominal injuries is becoming a rarer and rarer event. Angiography and a better scientific appreciation of which blunt solid organ injuries can be safely managed without intervention has improved the success rate of non-operative management. However evidence of significant abdominal injuries in the face of other concomitant injuries can create problems for the traumatologist.

The most commonly injured organs are the spleen and liver; however, small bowel and mesenteric injuries are becoming more common, especially with increasing seat belt use. Abdominal injuries are very vexing since our diagnostic tests, as good as they are, are not perfect. All trauma surgeons have had patients with completely negative abdominal CT scans, who 3 days into their stay become septic, are taken to OR, and found to have bowel injuries. Retrospective review of their original CTs is often unrevealing. It merely reinforces the importance of running toward problems that begin to present themselves, and re-evaluating patients and taking abnormalities and changes in condition seriously.

A thorough discussion of the management of abdominal injuries is well beyond the scope of this book. However, some central concepts should be part of the trauma center's ethos:

- A negative FAST or CT in a continually unstable patient requires re-evaluation and repeat imaging, or in some cases a trip to the OR.
- High-grade liver and spleen injuries with evidence of moderate to severe intra-abdominal hemorrhage require close observation. Even though prolonged bedrest (>3 days) is a concept not well supported by the literature, these patients are at the highest risk of deterioration. An old maxim is that "failure of non-operative management of liver injuries is a slow process, and failure of non-operative management of splenic injuries can be catastrophic." As we liberalize the management of lower grade solid organ injury, it is important to remember that people still die of liver and spleen injuries after they receive medical treatment, and this is avoidable.
- Hollow viscus injuries are the most difficult. As already stated, many have subtle findings, and in some, no findings on imaging. All major trauma patients have abdominal soreness (though patients with an isolated blunt small intestine injury are distinctive. They have an amazing amount of pain which should lead you to the diagnosis).

  - If the patient had abnormal initial imaging but no absolute indication for surgery (some intraperitoneal fluid, stranding, etc., but no definitive signs of hollow viscus injury) emergency repeat imaging with oral contrast is necessary at 6–8 hours as long as the patient's condition remains stable.
  - If the patient is unstable or has peritoneal signs, a trip to the OR is indicated. Some recommend laparoscopy in these instances; I do not. Injuries can be easy to miss, and the average laparoscopist is not competent to run the entire small bowel and inspect the entire colon. If you believe you can; then do so.
  - In the patient with an abnormal CT but no operative indications, keeping them in the hospital until they eat

and have a normal WBC is just safe practice. I will often check a lipase and amylase but repeat checks of these values are not well supported by the literature.

– DPL (diagnostic peritoneal lavage) is of mostly historical value at this time, and most current residents have never seen a DPL. But a DPL is an option in these patients with unclear findings.
– Patients with major abdominal and chest injuries belong on the trauma service and in the surgical ICU, no matter what other injuries they may have. That is why your SICU must be competent in severe head injury management.

Every trauma surgeon should be facile with abdominal injuries; however, some injuries can be so severe that consultation is warranted. I have called in hepatobiliary and transplant surgeons in the past for their opinion, as well as vascular surgery. This should not be an affront to the ego, and all should remember the patient is most important, and getting the best advice is critical.

However, if major bleeding is controlled, the patient should not be allowed to get cold and coagulopathic waiting for a specialist surgeon. Leave the abdomen open with or without packing and bring the specialist in with you when you bring the patient back for their second surgery.

Interventional radiology can often be lifesaving in major abdominal injuries to the liver and pelvis. I have brought IR in on many cases, and I believe this has improved our outcomes in especially difficult cases. Remember that you must always bring a critical care team with you to radiology in these cases and not leave the care of a complex patient in IR to the ED nursing staff or the IR nursing staff.

There is much more that could be said about abdominal injuries, but this book is more about how the trauma center system interacts with these patients, and less about the treatment of the injuries. There are several excellent books on the treatment of abdominal injuries (notably "Top Knife" by Ken

Mattox and Asher Hirshberg) [5]. The keys to managing major abdominal injuries in your system should be:

- Early notification
- Rapid diagnosis and movement through ED phase of care
- Blood availability and use
- OR availability
- IR capability and response
- Critical care capability

Major Spine

Major spine injuries are of course very significant to the individual but usually do not fall in the hyper-urgent realm. Spine injuries are obviously a major cause of morbidity, but in the vast majority of cases the workup is going to be completed before significant spine surgery occurs. There may be instances where the spine team will try to get the patient in traction or a halo in the emergency department, but lately our spine team has left these patients in a collar with spinal precautions and operated on them within 8 hours if it was an emergent issue.

The issue was spine injuries attributing hypotension to neurogenic shock when it is actually due to hypovolemic shock. You need to ensure that your clinicians always think of neurogenic shock as a diagnosis of exclusion after you've excluded thoracic abdominal and pelvic injuries as a cause of the patient's hypotension.

In my experience, the use of vasopressin agents in the emergency department usually should require experienced trauma attending input and should not be left up to trainees or ED providers. When you place an acute trauma patient on vasoactive agents in the early phases of care you need to be absolutely sure that you are not masking hypovolemic shock. If you mask hypotension with vasoactive agents, you will almost certainly have a patient with severe organ failure or death.

The proper workup to exclude spine injuries is the point of great argument among trauma surgeons and spine specialists. I will not try to detail those arguments here but if you examine our UVA trauma manual you will see that we are constantly revising our protocols for spinal evaluation based on the latest literature. An issue of spine evaluation is the fear of creating a patient with a lifelong disability when it could be avoided; however, we need to look at the actual literature to determine whether we are subjecting patients to too many tests and excessive immobilization when the chance of an injury that may require intervention is exceedingly small. In our manual we state "never be a cowboy with spine," but you can take this too far. Not all patients require complete spinal imaging CT scans, and MRIs, and you need to intelligently design a process for spinal evaluation that is logical and evidence-based.

Critically Ill Multiple Trauma Patient ("Big Crunch")

The last clinical discussion will focus on "the big crunch." These are the patients that Level I trauma centers were designed for, and these are the patients that test their capabilities to their limits. Unfortunately in this day and age, we are seeing "big crunches" in elderly patients adding even more complex dimensions of their care.

A "big crunch" is a patient that has multisystem injuries (chest, head, abdominal, pelvic, extremity, and spine injuries) associated with physiologic derangement and multiple overlapping critical priorities. While care of these patients can seem daunting, referring back to your ABCs and basic tenets of trauma care (airway control, treatment of hemo- and pneumothorax, rapid blood-oriented resuscitation for hypotensive patients, application of pelvic binders when needed, and rapid identification of critical abdominal, thoracic, and brain injuries).

The keys in these patients are clear thinking and having all the data at your fingertips. Not knowing the patient has a pneumothorax, or a suspected bowel injury, or lactic acidosis, or a small subdural hematoma can lead to incorrect decisions and bad outcomes. That is why when you have complex patients, you have to have an orderly process in your mind for what information you need before you make each critical decision.

As I said before, in critically ill patients, it is imperative to remove potentially dangerous variables from the equation. For instance, if the patient has thoracic, abdominal, head, and orthopedic injuries but is awake and talking, it is probably safe practice to go ahead and control that patient's airway. For patients with multiple injuries, it is often very difficult to get them through the radiologic evaluation and to move them from stretcher to table without significant pain control. In a patient where you are unsure of their volume status or that may be having continuing bleeding, sedation without invasive monitoring (such as an arterial line) and a controlled airway could lead to a catastrophic situation in radiology or during transport.

The ABCs are always critically important in these patients. Often, I will stand at the foot of the bed in a patient who we do not yet have under control, get the attention of the entire team, and go through the ABCs to ensure that we all believe we have these areas stabilized. For instance, we may be told by the nurse that she feels the blood pressures have been inaccurate, and thus we need to place an arterial line. We may hear from the respiratory therapist that the peak pressures on the ventilator are elevated. We may hear from the person at the head of the bed that there is a lot of blood in the ET tube, and they are having difficulty ventilating. In other words, you want all of these critical issues as stable as possible before leaving the trauma bay.

When you look at the priorities in these types of patients beyond the ABCs, the hierarchy is shock and brain injury, conditions that can kill in the next 2 hours, orthopedic issues that may threaten a limb, and finally identification of all injuries. It is important to keep this hierarchy in mind because you may often be pushed by orthopedics to take a patient with a horrible open tib/fib fracture to the operating room when you have placed a pressure monitor in the brain to ensure that the small subdural that you found on CT scan isn't causing intracranial hypertension. As a trauma surgeon you must keep the patient's best interest in mind and take specialty services desires to get their problem taken care of first as a second consideration behind insuring the patient is stable.

Transport

The process of moving critically ill trauma patients from their ED phase, to radiology, and then either back to the ED, or to OR, ICU, or interventional radiology can be fraught with danger. At this point, the patient is for the most part an unknown. The brain and cavities have not been thoroughly evaluated, and if your team is efficient, you may have moved through the ED phase in 15–20 minutes. You will evaluate the airway and make a decision about securing it; performed a FAST exam and obtained a chest x-ray and a pelvis x-ray. You will have drawn labs and possibly could have an arterial blood gas result back. You have also watched the patient for a short period of time to assess their stability.

At this point you need to complete the workup by obtaining head, cervical spine, and chest/abdomen and pelvis CT scans, and most likely an assortment of plain x-rays. In 90% of trauma patients, this transport will be safe, but in a small percentage, bad things can happen. These can include:

- Loss of airway
- Drop in blood pressure
- Oversedation
- Exacerbation of spine orthopedic injuries
- Other complications

Often the team that travels with the patient from the emergency department to radiology consists of an emergency department nurse, technician and possibly a respiratory therapist. However, at this point the patient is not really an emergency department patient but is much more similar to a critical care patient in the surgical ICU. While many emergency department nurses have some critical care experience, they rarely have equivalent experience to a full-time surgical ICU nurse. As a qualifier, some trauma centers do spend considerable effort to train their ED nurses to provide all necessary critical care needs. You need to evaluate your own center in this regard.

If the trauma center can arrange a system such that a SICU nurse can come down and accompany a critical trauma patient after leaving the emergency department that is often optimal. However, with staffing issues, this is not possible on a routine basis.

At the very least, members of the trauma team need to have the capability to recognize and intervene for life-threatening conditions during transport. This is not the medical student but needs to be an experienced PGY-1 or senior resident or nurse practitioner/physician's assistant.

The dangers inherent in patient transport following resuscitation have led to many standard practices in Level I trauma centers. These include ensuring that the patient has adequate IV access, ensuring that airway control is obtained in any patient where this is tenuous, and placing chest tubes in the emergency department for hemothoraces or pneumothoraces that are visible on the initial chest x-ray so these conditions do not worsen in radiology causing decompensation. While some of these measures may appear aggressive, your first priority in taking care of the injured patient is to prevent further harm. In addition, patients with multiple fractures and conditions requiring invasive intervention will be experiencing anxiety and severe pain. Sedating these patients with narcotics and benzodiazepines without securing their airway can be very dangerous. Therefore, in the critical multiple trauma patient, the patient with head injury, or the patient in shock, we will normally secure the airway with an endotracheal tube before leaving the trauma bay. Should it turn out that the patient has no injuries on radiologic evaluation and is beginning to wake up and follow commands, the patient can be taken back to the emergency department, safely extubated and sent to the acute care floor.

In many critical trauma patients, we elect to place large bore central venous catheters and arterial catheters. This will ensure that we have adequate access to handle any resuscitation situation and will also provide us with an accurate way of measuring the patient's blood pressure in real time so that we can intervene for any problems quickly. Many trauma surgeons know that using the noninvasive blood pressure cuff in a situation where you cannot directly observe the patient can lead to problems. These blood pressure cuffs tend to be inaccurate at the outside ranges of blood pressure (either very high or very low) thus making them less than useful in patients in shock.

During transport to radiology, the team should be planning the next phase of care for the patient, whether that be in the intensive care unit, the acute care floor, the operating room, or back in the emergency department for further treatment. It is always good practice in a critical trauma patient never to return to the emergency department once you have left. This allows the emergency department to clean the room and prepare for the next patient, to reclaim their staff, and it moves the patient into a critical care environment as rapidly as possible. For patients that have developed complex problems such as inability to ventilate effectively, refractory hypotension without an obvious source, or a degrading neurologic exam, often the best place for these patients is in an intensive care unit that regularly cares for seriously injured patients

Handoff of Care

One of the areas with the greatest risk of error is the handoff of care between teams and between units. This is because perishable critical information in the possession of the treating team can be forgotten, or not effectively transferred to the team that will begin to take care the patient. In the past, before electronic medical records, many people developed a system of writing down key information on the piece of paper and keeping in their pocket. They could then refer this piece of paper that would often have all the necessary presenting information, patient medical history, initial examination findings, lab values, and radiology findings to effectively transfer this information to the oncoming team. However, with the advent of electronic medical records, it requires somewhat more effort to log into a computer, find the patient record, and begin a detailed report of all of this information. Often this action comes after the patient has settled in whatever unit they are going to, and the physician has time to catch up on their paperwork and enter the data needed for the history and physical. The problem is that there is now a gap between the old paper system and the new electronic system such that there is no consistent standard work for recording critical information and effectively transferring it to the new care team.

There are many tools to try to improve the safety of handoff of care, but none have really gained widespread use. Many electronic medical record systems have notetaking capabilities and handoff reports that allow one team to communicate information to the next team; however, entering data in these reports can be time-consuming, and often cannot be done from a handheld device. This requires the practitioner to find a desktop computer, login, find the patient record, open relevant document, fill it in, and save it. As you can imagine, this process would take far more time than taking a notepad at your pocket and writing down the critical data. Therefore, it is important that the trauma system at least create standard work for the type of information that should be transferred between teams. The best system would be that the same practitioner team that handled the resuscitation the emergency department also handles the first 8 hours of care in the intensive care unit. However, most trauma centers do not function this way, and the emergency department resuscitation team is usually different than the ICU team. Below is our standard

SICU handoff of care checklist for postoperative patients and fresh trauma patients (Fig. 7.1).

It is strongly recommended that the trauma center develop simple checklists that each practitioner uses to relate critical information. It is also important to avoid making these checklists too detailed and too onerous, since they will not be used if that is the case. Experienced practitioners should sit

---

STBICU Admission HOC

Required for HOC: Primary Surgical MD, Anesthesia LIP, STBICU LIP, Bedside RN and RT

SURGERY
- [ ] Patient Name, MRN, and DOB
- [ ] Diagnosis
- [ ] Procedure / Technical Details
- [ ] Tubes/Drains
- [ ] Anticipated Course
- [ ] Hemodynamic Goals (including ICP, lumber drain)
- [ ] High Risk Meds (Vasoactive, anti-coags, steroids, etc)
- [ ] Transfusion Triggers
- [ ] Call Back Triggers
- [ ] Potential Problems

ANESTHESIA
- [ ] Allergies
- [ ] Relevant Past Medical History
- [ ] Unexpected Intra-op events, EBL
- [ ] Intubation (difficulty, ventilation issues)
- [ ] Plan for Extubation (collaborative decision)
- [ ] Vascular Access
- [ ] High Risk Meds (Hand off pumps to bedside RN)
- [ ] Total Blood Products Administered
- [ ] Blood Cooler (contents, expiration, return to BB?)
- [ ] Relevant Labs
- [ ] I/O in OR

ALL
- [ ] Questions / Concerns
- [ ] All remain present until HOC complete

FIGURE 7.1 Standard SICU handoff of care checklist

together in a room and decide what critical information is needed to properly intake of patient into the ICU, or the operating room, thus ensuring a measure of safety. Below I have included a typical checklist from our trauma manual (Fig. 7.2).

There will be situations where patients will have rapid decompensation during stages of transport. This can happen in the elevator, and a hallway, or upon entering the intensive care unit. It is important in these situations to rapidly evaluate the patient and not become angry or accusatory for the

☐ Call Trauma Alert if criteria met

☐ Large IV access

☐ If hypotensive, begin blood products and activate blood alert

☐ Rectal → (+) for high riding prostate or blood at meatus – NO Foley – call Urology

☐ Distal pulses

☐ Distal neuro exam

☐ Consider intubation for shock

☐ Check CXR

☐ FAST – positive and hypotensive – OR, normotensive – CT

☐ Binding device for pubic diastasis

☐ Check CT for BLUSH

☐ Open fracture – Tetanus and antibiotics

☐ Unstable or stable with large amount of hemorrhage or blush → call Interventional Radiology

☐ GU for hematuria

☐ Ortho to bedside

☐ ICU bed

☐ Critical trauma patient labs and notifications

☐ Consider binder for pubic diastasis

FIGURE 7.2 Trauma manual checklist for severe pelvic fracture

transporting team. "Life is dynamic" is a phrase I often use to remind people that a decompensating patient is often not the fault of any person but is merely the evolution of whatever process is going on. It is also another reason why it's important to run toward problems and intervene aggressively before problems become critical.

When a patient arrives in the condition that is not as advertised, it is vital to gather nurses and practitioners together immediately. Is often necessary in these situations to forgo some of the routine processes that occur upon transfer of patient to an ICU bed and to rewind the clock to a resuscitative mindset with focus on airway breathing and circulation. Once stabilization has occurred, then it is also vital for everyone to step back and go through a detailed handoff of care.

References

1. Meredith JW, Young JS, Bowling J, Roboussin D. Nonoperative management of blunt hepatic trauma: the exception or the rule? J Trauma. 1994;36:529–34.
2. Alton TB, Gee AO. Classifications in brief: young and burgess classification of pelvic ring injuries. Clin Orthop Relat Res. 2014;472(8):2338–42.
3. Cothren CC, Osborn PM, Moore EE, et al. Preperitoneal pelvic packing for hemodynamically unstable pelvic fractures: a paradigm shift. J Trauma. 2007;62:834–42.
4. Battle CE, Hutchings H, Lovett S, Boumara O, Jones S, et al. Predicting outcomes after blunt chest trauma: development and external validation of a new prognostic model. Crit Care. 2014;18(3):R98.
5. Hirshberg A, Mattox K. Top knife. Shrewsbury: TFM Publishing; 2005.

Chapter 8
First 8 Hours

Initial ICU Assessment

Preparation and Handoff

We have previously discussed the importance of a thorough and efficient handoff of care. This is extremely important in handing off the patient to the ICU team. We have a fairly regimented script for this handoff that is shown previously. We use this script for both the transfer of a trauma patient and the transfer of a postoperative patient from the OR. We demand that the on-call SICU or trauma ICU (TICU) resident, the anesthesia resident, the nurse, the respiratory therapist, and charge nurse be present for these handoffs. If you are in a center where your trauma resuscitation and ICU teams are one in the same, then there is no need for detailed handoff between physician teams, but there is still a need for handoff with the nursing staff that the physicians should be present for.

It is also vital during this handoff and in preparing for the patient's arrival to have some idea of what the plan is for the next 8 hours. Is the patient going back for more radiological

© Springer Nature Switzerland AG 2020
J. S. Young, *Trauma Centers*,
https://doi.org/10.1007/978-3-030-34607-2_8

studies? Is the patient going to the operating room? Is the patient going to interventional radiology? This will allow the nurses to ensure that they have adequate staff and equipment to take road trips with these patients. Adequate staffing is often a major obstacle in trauma critical care because common complex trips off unit are unpredictable, and thus it is difficult for unit managers to properly staff for the contingency of multiple critically ill trauma patients.

ABC's, Hemodynamics, and Resuscitation

Obviously, there is a wide range of criticality among trauma ICU admissions, but in all admissions, it is important to accurately measure and assess the patient's hemodynamics and their status with regard to resuscitation and acidosis. There should already be initial lab studies from the emergency department as well as blood pressure and pulse trends. As I said previously in the most critically ill patients, we will often place an arterial catheter to have real-time measurement of blood pressure. It is also critical to continue to evaluate the ABC's of patients since problems can creep in during the late emergency department phase and during the transport phase. Another area of danger is when the patient is in a specialty procedure area for an extended period of time between the emergency department stay and the intensive care unit.

As is routine in almost every ICU when the patient arrives, respiratory therapy will assess the status of the airway and breathing. In the intubated patient, they will assess cuff pressure, depth of the endotracheal tube, and breath sounds and will almost always obtain arterial blood gas measurement in any intubated patient. At this point, in many situations, sedation and paralytics have begun to wear off, and patients will begin to fight the ventilator and become agitated. It is vital when this occurs to make a rational assessment of whether the patient can be extubated and not rush into this decision.

Often patients will become agitated when they awaken with the tube in the back of the throat, but their respiratory status precludes extubation. You will often have staff who push you to remove the endotracheal tube as patients wake up, and it is vital to resist this urge and continue to gather data such as a chest x-ray and arterial blood gas measurements to ensure that the patient can survive without ventilatory support.

The nursing staff will assess the status of the patient's intravenous lines, dressings, catheters, and tubes. They will also gather information on the status of the family and contact information and inquire whether the family has arrived at the hospital yet and whether they have been spoken with. It is often the case that families will be directed to the intensive care unit waiting area before the patient even arrives in the ICU, leaving the unit staff confused as to which patient they are concerned about. This is another reason to book your room in the intensive care unit as soon as you know that the patient will not be able to be cared for outside of the critical care area. This way the nurses can communicate the current location of the patient to the family and give them a realistic estimation of when the patient will arrive in the ICU.

The routine actions on arrival in the ICU will be a fresh sampling of venous blood for hematology and chemistry measurement. It is also important to obtain a lactic acid sample at this time. For any ventilated patient or any patient with significant thoracic injuries who may not be ventilated, an arterial blood gas is prudent. All of these labs should be sent STAT and should be followed up upon quickly.

Obviously, any airway issues that become evident must be dealt with immediately, which is a key reason to have doctors, nurses, and respiratory therapists at the bedside on the arrival of the patient. The patency of the airway should be immediately assessed since it may have changed since the patient was first evaluated. It is also important not to overreact agitation in this phase with heavy sedation since the agitation may be a sign of shock or respiratory insufficiency.

Plans for the Next 4–8 Hours

At this point, after ensuring that the ABC's are intact and the patient is stable, you should begin to think about and plan for the next 4 hours. This will include whether you will wean the patient to extubation, whether you will allow the patient to go for orthopedic or other specialty surgery, whether neurosurgery needs to place a bolt or ventricular drain, whether you need to begin intracranial hypertension treatment, etc.

With regard to extubation, we often feel that if the patient arrives in the intensive care in the evening, we would prefer to wait until the following morning to extubate unless the patient is wide awake with minimal ventilator support. The reasons for this are the decrease in staffing at night in the ICUs and decreased attending coverage. Usually this will only entail another 12 hours of ventilator support which should cause very little morbidity. Also, during this time many patients require trips to radiology for further studies, and these are safer with the airway controlled. Often the operative plans have not been decided upon in those first few hours in the ICU and is suboptimal to extubate a patient and have them re-intubated for surgery a few hours later. At this time it is also important to plan out road trips for repeat head CT scans, MRI studies, or other diagnostic studies. But if the patient looks great and all parameters point toward extubation, go ahead with it.

The patient's acid-base and acidosis status needs to be assessed at this time. We do this through examination of lactic acid values and bicarbonate values. You should have an initial lactic acid value from the patient's arrival in the emergency department and at least one more before arrival in the intensive care unit. This will allow you to identify a trend in the patient's acidosis if present. If you see the patient may still have an abnormal lactic acid but it is dropping sharply into the normal range, it is not unreasonable to allow the patient to go for orthopedic procedures immediately. However, if lactic acid values are high and not dropping, or rising, it is not prudent to allow the patient to go to the OR for any other procedure than ones that are lifesaving. Significant blood loss in the operating room from orthopedic procedures when the patient is already acidotic can have a devastating effect on morbidity and mortality. This is especially important in the elderly patients with serious comorbidities. Frequent lab studies for the first 12 hours in the intensive care unit are important in order to identify any problems and trends. At this time orthopedics may want to place femoral traction or tibial traction plans, neurosurgery may wish to place spine stabilization devices, and face surgeons may want to do a calmer repair of facial lacerations and injuries. All of this can be allowed since the patient will not need to move from the room or from the critical care environment.

Occult Hypoperfusion

Our trauma group has written extensively on occult hypoperfusion and its effect on outcome [1–3]. We feel persistent lactic acidosis is an important predictor of respiratory and multiple organ failure. Our goal is to correct all acidosis within 12 hours through resuscitation or bleeding control. If the patient's lactic acidosis persists past 12 hours, echocardiogram, Swan Ganz catheter placement, or noninvasive perfusion monitoring should be considered. The patient's urine output during this time is also of vital importance. If the patient has evidence of occult hypoperfusion as well as oliguria, this demands rapid intervention to prevent renal failure and cascading organ failure. It is important not to correct lactic acidosis through administration of sodium bicarbonate. Resuscitation is the cure for lactic acidosis, blood is superior to crystalloid as a resuscitation fluid, and persistent acidosis needs to bring up the possibility of continued bleeding from identified or occult injuries.

Elderly patients with restricted cardiac reserve can often have difficulty correcting their acidosis on their own. This is especially true in patients with reduced cardiac output. In these patients it is not unusual to need to start some pressor or inotropic support. Clinicians need to be careful not to use a pressor that will worsen cardiac performance by increasing systemic vascular resistance. This increases afterload and puts more strain on a heart that may be struggling to meet perfusion needs. We need to add vasopressor drips in less than 7% of our patients with occult hypoperfusion. The other 93% will be corrected by resuscitation and bleeding control. Perhaps the most dangerous part of using drugs such as norepinephrine in a fresh trauma patient is that it will falsely elevate the blood pressure masking underlying hypovolemia and possibly significant bleeding as its cause. Anytime a patient is on a norepinephrine drip in the first 24 hours after trauma admission, the clinician must be extremely suspicious that there is an underlying problem that needs treatment.

Respiratory Failure

The scope of treatment for respiratory failure is far beyond this book; however, it is important to remember some basic principles. Trauma patients are often intubated for a variety of reasons including protection during the diagnostic phase, agitation, inability to treat the patient, true respiratory failure, shock, etc. For those patients who had normal mental status for intubation and a normal head CT scan (or CT scan with only minimal findings) who also will not require surgery in the next 12–24 hours should have an arterial blood gas drawn, repeat chest x-ray, and a discussion with respiratory therapy to begin the wean the patient off ventilatory support with the expectation that they be extubated in a short period of time. For those patients who were intubated for hypoxia, hypercarbia, and shock, early weaning to extubation is probably unwise. It is far safer to allow an 8- to 12-hour time course to elapse to ensure that the patient is well resuscitated, that there is no evidence of ongoing bleeding, and that they don't have structural defects in their chest or lungs that will cause them to fail extubation.

From our own experience we feel it is vital to obtain real data before making decisions regarding extubation and weaning. A daily chest x-ray and a chest x-ray after any period of respiratory decompensation are necessary. At least daily arterial blood gas, and a repeat determination after major changes in ventilator support, or at least when the patient reaches minimal ventilator settings are mandatory under our guidelines. A common problem is transient changes in oxygen saturation that lead to overreaction on the part of respiratory therapy. This leads to seemingly small changes in ventilatory support that over time become large changes. This includes increasing the patient's PEEP in response to an oxygen saturation of less than 92% or a large increase in the inspired oxygen concentration for the same indication. Once the patient's ventilatory support has been significantly increased, it becomes harder to wean them efficiently. This is why we expect that no great changes in ventilatory support will be made for single episodes of low oxygen saturation. When these episodes occur, it is far more likely that the patient has begun to awaken and fight the ventilator and thus is not ventilating optimally. Either placing the patient on continuous positive airway pressure (CPAP), or providing reasonable sedation will correct most of these problems. Often this occurs during turning of the patient when previously poorly perfused and injured areas of the lung now have increased blood flow. Usually this will resolve on turning the patient back supine and waiting a few minutes.

Neurologic

The treatment of traumatic brain injury is unfortunately variable and without therapies that have strong evidence of efficacy [4]. In our experience the best predictor of the patient's recovery from traumatic brain injury was their mental status immediately after the traumatic event. A patient with a GCS of three when found by EMS makes us extremely concerned about long-term recovery. Patients that are fighting or agitated when found by EMS but not clearly following commands will often have a better outcome, and the best outcomes are found in those patients that were merely disoriented or intubated for reasons other than coma.

It is generally accepted that current therapy for traumatic brain injury includes measurement of intracranial pressure for prudent indications, inducement of hyponatremia in the range of 150–155 mg/dl, achievement of a partial carbon dioxide concentration of between 33 and 36 mmHg, sedation to reduce the neurons use of oxygen, elevation of the head of the bed if possible, avoidance of compression of the jugular veins, and of course early surgical intervention for intracranial mass lesions that are amenable to evacuation.

Orthopedic Injuries

The saving of life comes over the saving of limb in all cases. Thus, the patient with critical injuries to the cardiac, respiratory, or neurologic systems needs treatment and stabilization of those injuries prior to orthopedic fixation. Our own studies found that in orthopedic fixation patient, persistent lactic acidosis increases the rate of complications [3]. But there is abundant data that early fixation allows early ambulation and a decrease in pulmonary complications. Discussion with the orthopedic traumatologist on call as to the urgency of operative treatment is important in the first 8 hours after arrival in the critical care unit. This will allow you to make a plan for the next several days as to when the patient will need to go to the operating room, or it will allow you to explain to the orthopedist that a trip to the operating room in the near future is not possible and they will need to look for ways to stabilize fractures at the bedside. In addition, it is important to discuss the expected blood loss from these procedures so that the patient is properly prepared for surgery. In our experience patients that leave the ICU for major orthopedic operations should return to the ICU even if they are extubated in the operating room and appear to be stable. After reviewing their condition for a few hours, they can be transferred out. In truth, families may be the most concerned about broken arms and legs, and it is imperative that the traumatologist discusses issues from most likely to threaten life to those least likely to do it. It is important that families understand the priorities that are necessary in planning treatment.

We use a daily checklist shown as in Fig. 8.1. We use this checklist on rounds to ensure that we are covering all critical problems with corrective actions. We go through this after the presentation and before moving in the next patient. It does not matter whether the nurse, the resident, or the attending goes through the checklist as long as each item is reviewed. It is also reasonable to only bring up items on the checklist that

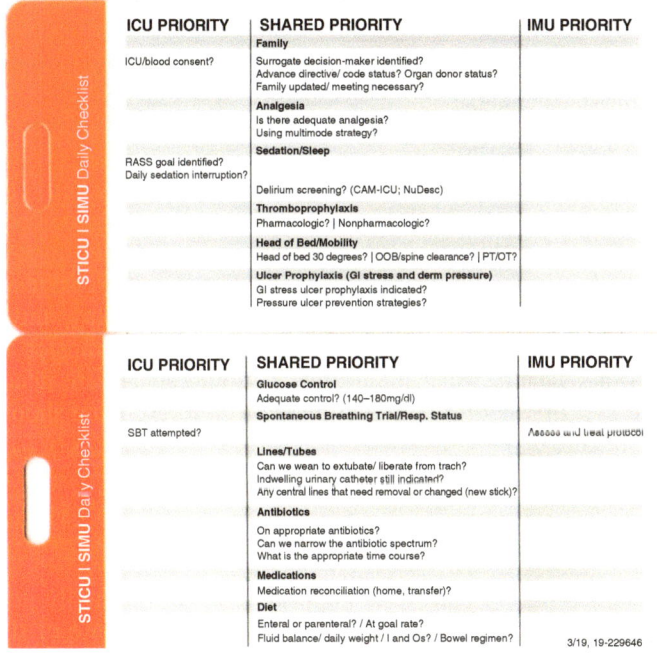

STICU I SIMU Daily Checklist	ICU PRIORITY	SHARED PRIORITY	IMU PRIORITY
		Family	
	ICU/blood consent?	Surrogate decision-maker identified? Advance directive/ code status? Organ donor status? Family updated/ meeting necessary?	
		Analgesia Is there adequate analgesia? Using multimode strategy?	
	RASS goal identified? Daily sedation interruption?	**Sedation/Sleep**	
		Delirium screening? (CAM-ICU; NuDesc)	
		Thromboprophylaxis Pharmacologic? | Nonpharmacologic?	
		Head of Bed/Mobility Head of bed 30 degrees? | OOB/spine clearance? | PT/OT?	
		Ulcer Prophylaxis (GI stress and derm pressure) GI stress ulcer prophylaxis indicated? Pressure ulcer prevention strategies?	

STICU I SIMU Daily Checklist	ICU PRIORITY	SHARED PRIORITY	IMU PRIORITY
		Glucose Control Adequate control? (140–180mg/dl)	
	SBT attempted?	**Spontaneous Breathing Trial/Resp. Status**	Assess and treat protocol
		Lines/Tubes Can we wean to extubate/ liberate from trach? Indwelling urinary catheter still indicated? Any central lines that need removal or changed (new stick)?	
		Antibiotics On appropriate antibiotics? Can we narrow the antibiotic spectrum? What is the appropriate time course?	
		Medications Medication reconciliation (home, transfer)?	
		Diet Enteral or parenteral? / At goal rate? Fluid balance/ daily weight / I and Os? / Bowel regimen?	3/19, 19-229646

Figure 8.1 Surgical trauma ICU daily checklist

were not covered and not go through every item in every patient. We have found that the checklist has improved our adherence to guidelines and has prevented errors. Most commonly these errors have involved delayed initiation of oral feeding, delayed mobilization, and delayed initiation of deep venous thrombosis (DVT) prophylaxis.

Transfer to Acute Care or Step-Down

As a patient's condition improves, plans will be made to move them to a lower level of care, either an intermediate care unit or the acute care floor. During this time between admission to the ICU and the discussion of transfer, the duties of the critical care team are to surveil for complications, to intervene on significant findings, to work with multiple specialty teams to plan out treatment, to keep the family informed the patient's progress, and to make the patient as comfortable as reasonably possible.

As the patient is weaning from the ventilator and any significant infusions move toward taking medications and food orally, a plan should be made for moving to a lower level of care. A plan for DVT prophylaxis, advancement of oral feedings, activity, physical therapy, occupational therapy, and a discussion of whether the patient will require transfer to another facility when the critical care and acute care needs are met or whether they will be allowed to go home should be begun.

Safety

A strong safety culture is imperative to an optimally performing trauma center. In our trauma manual, one of the first statements on one of the first pages is that we run toward problems and not away from them and that you will never get in trouble for aggressively ruling out a potentially serious problem. We will review some patient safety issues.

DVT Prophylaxis

We ask about DVT prophylaxis on every single patient every day. If specialty services are denying our request to begin prophylaxis, we have a discussion with them on a daily basis as to when we can expect to be able to begin prophylaxis and what prophylaxis we can use. As the literature has supported low-molecular-weight heparin as the most effective preventative measure for DVT and pulmonary embolism, this is our preferred medication. Unfractionated heparin is generally considered to be less effective but better than no chemical prophylaxis. As is been reported in many studies, mechanical prophylaxis has poor compliance, and the devices are often found hanging from the end of the bed instead of on the patient's extremities. We do order mechanical prophylaxis on all patients where it is possible, but we feel chemical prophylaxis with low-molecular-weight heparin is our standard for DVT prevention.

We consider a certain category of patients very high-risk thromboembolism and DVT. These include patients with lower extremity fractures, pelvic fractures, severe head injury, and spinal cord injury or prolonged immobilization. In these patients we are very nervous about delaying chemical prophylaxis and will often have a frank discussion with the family and/or the patient about placement of a vena cava filter. All filters we place are removable, and a process should be in place to remove the filter once the risk period has passed. We place far fewer filters today than we have in the past in response to several studies showing that prophylactic filter placement does not improve outcomes. But we still place filters in the following patients:

- Documentation of deep femoral thrombosis in a patient who was on full chemical prophylaxis
- Documentation of pulmonary embolism in a patient who was on full chemical prophylaxis
- Evidence of a life-threatening pulmonary embolism
- Discovery of a DVT or pulmonary embolism in a patient where effective chemical treatment is not possible

Infection Surveillance

Infections are a major cause of morbidity and mortality in trauma patients. Early intervention and appropriate intervention for bacterial infection improve outcome. However, many trauma patients, due to the amplified immune response, have fevers and occasionally leukocytosis. In addition, patients with multiple orthopedic injuries, facial injuries, abdominal injuries, and thoracic injuries are all prone to secondary infection.

In distinction to this is the rise of resistant bacteria with the overuse of antibiotics. The trauma service has to develop a process for infection surveillance and treatment that walks a middle line between overuse of antibiotics and delays in intervention. In our center during the first 48 hours, a fever will warrant a physical exam and a chest x-ray but usually no other diagnostic studies. Unless of course their injuries put them in a far higher risk of infection (open orthopedic fractures, large bowel injuries, etc.). Rising white count in these first 48 hours can merely be indicative of the stress response and not bacterial infection. We take several measures to prevent infection. These include changing of all central venous and arterial catheters within the first 12 hours of admission if they were placed in the emergency room or a referring hospital. While some of these lines could have been put under sterile conditions, we assume that they were not. In addition, we look for aspiration vigorously and perform bedside swallowing evaluations on all critical care patients. Patients who fail this will go on to a formal speech pathology swallowing evaluation.

All wounds must be carefully examined, and any evidence of purulence needs to be addressed. As care progresses past 48 hours, leukocytosis and fever or focal changes in the chest x-ray will warrant sputum, blood, and occasionally urine cultures, although we do not perform urine cultures routinely. My philosophy for diagnosing pulmonary infections is to talk to respiratory therapy about the character of the sputum and to perform aggressive bronchoscopy for significant changes in the chest x-ray. I also believe that sputum cultures should be gathered during any bronchoscopy. This is personal preference and the literature in this area is dynamic.

For life-threatening potential bacterial infections (leukocytosis or fever associated with increasing organ dysfunction, hypotension, or multiple organ dysfunction), we will often obtain cultures and simultaneously begin broad-spectrum antibiotic treatment. This treatment is of a limited duration (usually 72 hours) unless bacterial cultures are positive. As in many trauma centers, we have a pharmacist as part of our team, and we look to this team member to guide our antibiotic therapy when we have positive cultures. We try to give the most focused antibiotic therapy possible for the shortest duration. As we will discuss in the performance improvement chapters, antibiotic choices and durations that seem to be outside of generally accepted practice by specialty surgeons will be examined, and we will try to reach a consensus that is consistent with current literature.

The bottom line is to act aggressively to identify a source of infection, treat empirically if severe sepsis is feared, target antibiotic therapy based on cultures, and use the least antibiotics necessary for the least amount of time.

Nutrition

Providing nutrition to trauma and surgical patients is essential. We try to feed the gut as soon as possible after injury. Centers should avoid the use of total parenteral nutrition (TPN) if at all possible due to the infection risk and possibility of hepatic dysfunction with long-term use.

Aspiration is also a major cause of morbidity and occasionally mortality in trauma centers. As the age of trauma patients increases, patients with subclinical aspiration at home are often treated. We have undertaken a strategy of simple screening, followed by bedside nursing swallow evaluation. If the patient fails the bedside test, a formal evaluation is done by speech pathology. Should they fail that a gastrostomy tube is often placed if acceptable to the patient or family.

Clinical nutritionists should be a part of the trauma team and either round concurrently or report their recommendations to the team on a daily basis.

Rehabilitation

Rehabilitation and post-acute care are critical factors in optimal recovery. There are some centers where a physiatrist rounds with the trauma team or sees certain categories of patients daily. Physical and occupational therapy evaluations are critical and should be timely.

Discharge and Follow-up

It is important that patients are given clear instructions for discharge (diet, activity, medications) and confirmed follow-up. In our clinic, our primary purpose is to insure that patients are being properly followed by all relevant services. Weaning from narcotics is also important, and the discussion of duration and depth of pain control should be done on discharge and again at every visit.

References

1. Blow O, Magliore L, Claridge JA, Butler K, Young JS. The golden hour and the silver day: detection and correction of occult hypoperfusion within 24 hours improves outcome from major trauma. J Trauma. 1999;47:964–9.
2. Claridge JA, Crabtree TD, Pelletier SJ, Butler K, Sawyer RG, Young JS. Persistent occult hypoperfusion is associated with a significant increase in infection rate and mortality in major trauma patients. J Trauma. 2000;48:8–14.

3. Crowl AC, Young JS, Kahler DM, Claridge JA, Chrzanowski DS, Pomphrey M. Occult hypoperfusion is associated with increased morbidity in patients undergoing early femur fracture fixation. J Trauma. 2000;48:260–7.
4. Brain Trauma Foundation. Guidelines for the management of severe traumatic brain injury. 2016. Braintrauma.org, https://braintrauma.org/uploads/03/12/Guidelines_for_Management_of_Severe_TBI_4th_Edition.pdf.

Part III
Performance Improvement

Chapter 9
Structure

As stated in the previous chapters, a strong performance improvement program is the key element of a high-performing trauma center. There are many different configurations for a performance improvement program (PI), and centers differ in their basic processes. In general, the trauma medical director should be leading the PI program. This includes how cases are chosen for examination, what sort of analyses are done, how corrective action plans are constructed, how feedback is executed with liaisons and patient care units, and determining that the loop closures have been implemented. The trauma program manager has an equally important role in that they will be most often the hands-on person dealing with case follow-up and loop closure.

Many programs are now employing a performance improvement coordinator. This is usually an experienced nurse from either the ICU or the ED who has spent some time working on patient safety and quality. In many programs the PI coordinator is given latitude in setting up filters, choosing cases for higher tier examination, coordinating multidisciplinary performance improvement meetings, and handling communications regarding PI cases.

© Springer Nature Switzerland AG 2020   127
J. S. Young, *Trauma Centers*,
https://doi.org/10.1007/978-3-030-34607-2_9

The trauma registry is also an essential part of an effective PI program. If data gathering and data integrity are poor, then no matter how high the quality of the rest of the program is, it will be working with faulty information. In most ACS-verified centers, the registrar will also be responsible for submitting data to TQIP (ACS trauma quality improvement program). Since TQIP is the only widely accepted benchmarking system for trauma in the USA, inaccurate data entry can lead to inaccurate benchmarking. The trauma registry coordinator or the lead trauma registrar should be well trained and have completed the basic trauma registry courses provided throughout the country. They should be responsible for ensuring data accuracy in the registry and among the other registry staff.

Specialty liaisons need to be thoroughly integrated into the PI program so that assignment of cases, completion of analysis, implementation of corrective actions, and loop closure in their specialties are done expeditiously. Also the other core trauma surgeons should be intimately involved with the PI process and should also be involved with mortality case review from other surgeons in the program.

We will discuss this in detail in subsequent chapters, but a functioning PI program must:

- Audit overall performance with regard to
    - Mortality
    - Complications
    - Efficiency
    - Errors and near misses
    - Performance by severity of injury
    - Length of stay
    - Response to activations
    - Surgical specialty response
    - Trauma surgeon response to highest level activations
    - Delays in treatment
    - And other areas as determined by the program

There is no magic number of metrics to look at, and some programs can do excellent work with few filters by drilling deeply into each case. Other can be ineffective because they look at everything and delve into nothing. An immature program should probably pick 5–10 metrics to examine, and this can be decreased as they become more facile with PI. Mature programs often will choose one metrics for a year or so, determine that they are performing adequately, and move on to look deeply into another area while monitoring the former process. This is not a substitute for a robust dashboard where the program can monitor basic measurements of performance. These are specific problems that require concentrated effort.

Naturally, the structure of the PI program should allow the TPM and TMD to maintain situational awareness of significant problems and insure that they are being acted upon. The problem with following too many processes is that the program can get lost and not improve anything. Alternately the problem with only looking at a narrow amount of filters is that the program can get tunnel vision and think they are doing well when there are serious problems. It is also critical that the program has a method for frontline personnel to report problems. Often the frontline nurse or technician sees problems before they would ever reach the level of the TMD. Frontline staff should be encouraged to report issues up through their unit managers or directly to the trauma program. In my own program, frontline personnel opened fruitful areas of investigation by bringing our attention to problems that we could not see.

As we will discuss later, representatives from clinical areas, lab, blood bank, EMS, prehospital communication, emergency management, and specialty liaisons are critical links in identifying problems and implementing solutions. There should be forums where all of these contributors to the care of the injured patient can meet together and discuss patient care. At the least the program should demonstrate that they are receptive to concerns and will provide those who report issues with feedback to demonstrate the program is concerned and is investigating the issue.

PI meetings should be held regularly with mandatory representation from key stakeholders. Frequent absences may warrant discussion with the department chair of area administrator to insure that someone who is interested in the care of the injured is involved in the PI process. It is critical for the TPM or PI director to insure that these meetings are collegial and any interpersonal problems are dealt with outside of the view of the entire group. Sensitive issues related to peers should first be discussed in small groups to avoid embarrassment. Then the findings and corrective actions can be brought to the larger group.

In conclusion process comes from structure and structure control process. If the trauma center PI program is poorly structured, it can only move forward through heroic effort, which often leads to burnout and is unsustainable in the long term. Young programs should not be reticent to visit mature established programs and learn from them. No program should have to "reinvent the wheel" with regard to PI. There are literally dozens of trauma centers that do this well, and their structure should be integrated or even copied.

Chapter 10
What Is the Purpose of PI?

Philosophy

The purpose of PI is to improve care. In order to do this, you have to create a culture of safety. A culture of safety involves everyone who touches the patient. All of these professionals must come to work every day with the philosophy that no patient will get harmed under their watch. There are always instances where injury is unavoidable, but everyone must do everything within their power to ensure the patient's course is smooth. In order to do this, you have to create a "no-blame" environment. What that means is that staff must feel confident that if they report a problem, there will not be retribution. And they also must be confident that any report will be treated confidentially. Probably the most important is that all staff members must be receptive to constructive criticism and must be willing to accept changes in the process of care and improve outcomes. Performance improvement programs should not be hostile, or participants will cover up issues that could be critical to high-quality care. The entire trauma center executive staff (trauma medical director, trauma program manager, trauma registrar coordinator, trauma PI coordinator, and specialty liaisons) should work as a team to improve care.

© Springer Nature Switzerland AG 2020
J. S. Young, *Trauma Centers*,
https://doi.org/10.1007/978-3-030-34607-2_10

We do not always know if the proposed change in the standard work will be beneficial, but it is the process that is important, that is:

- Identifying something that is in need of improvement or that has injured the patient
- Examining it thoroughly with input from the frontline staff
- Identifying a future state where the problem no longer exists
- Analyzing the data to understand the issue
- Creating countermeasures to improve the process
- Following up to insure that your changes are being followed and that the desired effect on outcomes has occurred

Trauma has always been ahead of other inpatient areas in performance improvement in that from the first designation manuals, performance improvement was considered to be the most important feature of the well-functioning program. You could say that only since the 1999 Institute of Medicine report "to err is human" have hospitals jumped with both feet on the quality bandwagon, whereas trauma centers were doing this 15 years prior to that.

Data

Medicine has often suffered from a dearth of information that is accurate, relevant, and risk-adjusted to gauge performance. Only in the last decade or so have reliable benchmarking systems come into common use. There is a phrase "you can't manage what you can't measure" that does apply here. However, in many cases, we have to deal with the best data available, and sometimes this is not properly risk-adjusted. At the very least, every trauma center should be able to benchmark itself against itself, meaning that they can track their outcomes for certain populations of patients from year to year, track their adherence to guidelines and standard work, and track common complications and other processes of care. While their performance may not meet the top deciles in a national benchmarking program, all any program can do is strive to get better every year.

Scope

In its most basic form, performance improvement must monitor the care that is provided in the trauma center throughout the entire continuum of care. It cannot solely focus on inpatient care in that if it does, it will miss issues that involve EMS and aeromedical services. It also must complete the circle of care by having some knowledge of long-term outcomes of critically injured patients. The usual process is that the PI program will create a variety of filters in order to choose cases for further examination. At its most simple, every center must examine patient who died in the trauma center. Then programs have some latitude to choose other patient care filters. These can include unplanned extubation, time to splenectomy, time to craniotomy, time to open fracture treatment, time to femur and tibia fixation, time to antibiotic administration and open fractures, and time to beginning of interventional radiology procedures, ICP bolt placement rates for severe head injury, etc. While many of these filters are mandated by the American College of Surgeons, the program is free to choose other filters. These filters do not need to be permanent and could be implemented based on a single case or series of cases, and then closed to move onto another area of focus.

Opportunities for Improvement

Opportunities for improvements (OFIs) arc the basic unit of PI action. OFIs can take several forms. They can be personnel issues that hinder performance, lack of readily accessible equipment, medical errors, laboratory errors, blood bank issues, etc. OFIs provide PI programs with a core issue to analyze, define a desired future state, create countermeasures, implement change, and monitor for improvement. The terms I have used here are used in many performance improvement systems, but all quality techniques focus around PDSA (plan, do, study, act). Find a problem, design and implement a solution, study the effect of the solution, and then change and adapt as needed.

Examples of OFIs include the following:

- Delayed availability of an operating room for an emergency operation
- Delayed availability of blood products
- Delayed reporting of critical laboratory values
- Lack of venous thromboembolism prophylaxis when no contraindications exist in a high-risk patient
- Lack of follow-up of critical vital sign changes
- Poor communication between caregivers resulting in patient harm

Chapter 11
Event Analysis

We will take one of these OFIs I have listed and provide examples of the type of analysis that is expected.

- Delayed availability of blood products

  - Initial impression

    A patient with hypotension and evidence of bleeding from an unstable pelvic fracture did not receive blood within 60 minutes of the order being received by the blood bank.

  - Further data gathering

    Instead of placing the order through the routine pathways, some unknown person in the emergency department called up to the blood bank, spoke to a technician, and said they needed O negative blood for the trauma activation in the ED.

    The blood bank technician states that they called back to the ED for further information but were unable to reach someone who could provide patient data. Thus, they were unable to release the blood products.

    After 30 minutes the ED called the blood bank and was told the blood could not be released without a proper order; the order was placed through the proper process, and the blood arrived soon thereafter.

© Springer Nature Switzerland AG 2020
J. S. Young, *Trauma Centers*,
https://doi.org/10.1007/978-3-030-34607-2_11

- Analysis

  The hospital has an emergency blood release process where a form is signed by a physician taking care of the patient and brought to the blood bank, and four units of uncrossmatched blood is released.

  During the resuscitation, the physician called out "we need uncrossmatched blood." Someone trying to be helpful called the blood bank and yelled back into the trauma room that "the blood was ordered." This person was not aware of the emergency release process and was trying to help.

  The ED does not have a solid system for educating all team members about the emergency blood release process. In fact, after questioning, the TPM finds that most ED staff are not aware of the form, where it is, or the process of obtaining blood from the blood bank using the form.

At this point prior to creating corrective actions, the PI team needs to call in frontline people from ED, trauma, and blood bank to discuss the current process. Is it working if most ED staff were unaware of it? Do we need a simpler process? Should blood automatically be delivered to the trauma bay for certain types of patients? Where does a massive transfusion protocol (MTP) fit into these situations? Should an MTP have been activated?

- Discussion and creation of corrective actions

  - The frontline team with the PI team feels the current process is too cumbersome. The form takes several minutes to fill out and asks for information that is not available to anyone other than the nurse in the trauma bay.
  - The team felt there are situations where several units of blood may be needed, but that the MTP would be overkill and would lead to the wastage of blood products in many cases.

- In discussion with blood bank, it is decided to place a blood refrigerator in the trauma bay that is stocked with four units of O negative blood. This blood can be accessed by anyone on the trauma team. Before implementation the PI staff contacts centers that have a blood refrigerator in the ED to learn of pitfalls and optimal processes.
- The blood refrigerator is installed and the staff is educated. It is decided that an alarm is placed on the door of the refrigerator, and when opened, the blood bank is immediately notified. This allows them to inquire if further blood products are needed and notifies them that the refrigerator should be restocked.

- Auditing

  - For 6 months, the blood bank reports all instances where blood was removed from the refrigerator for use in trauma patients the day after it is used. The TPM or PI coordinator then examines the case and determines if the process is working as expected.
  - If no changes are needed, the auditing is stopped, and examination of the process will only occur if an issue arises.

Chapter 12
Regulatory Requirements

One of the problems with the head start that trauma centers had with performance improvement was that hospitals had to catch up. This means that many of the processes the trauma centers were using for decades were new to hospitals. This included thorough examination of mortality, identification of near misses, identification of some optimal care, event analysis and corrective action.

I was the chief quality officer for a major academic medical center for 9 years after I was the director of the trauma center for 10 years. On the hospital side, the entire process of examination of mortality and patient harm was at a very nascent phase. We had to build the process from nothing. We had to identify data sources, figure out how to find out what patients died in the hospital the previous day, what information we need from their chart, decide what information was necessary from the caregivers, decide how to bring these cases together for discussion, figure out how to create corrective action plans, and then implement these plans and provide follow-up. These are the types of activities that

© Springer Nature Switzerland AG 2020
J. S. Young, *Trauma Centers*,
https://doi.org/10.1007/978-3-030-34607-2_12

trauma centers have been doing for quite a while. Nationally, the Joint Commission initiated mandatory processes for all hospitals including the identification of sentinel events and other reporting processes. Even now trauma centers and hospitals have difficulty integrating their trauma and hospital performance improvement systems since they both run independently. One of the factors that we have begun to look at on ACS site visits is how the trauma program is bringing what they learn to the hospital and is the hospital bringing what they learn to the trauma program. However, this is often difficult because the trauma PI program is usually well-established and the hospital PI program is usually at an earlier phase.

Basically, the criteria that guide PI come from state trauma designation manuals, the ACS optimal resources document, and the Joint Commission [1]. I will not go into detail in any of these here since all of these documents are available. But they tend to revolve around a formalized structure with a leader, a formalized data gathering process, analysis process, scheduled meetings under the PI umbrella where frank discussions can be made, decision-making on the severity of harm, countermeasures, corrective action plan implementation, and auditing and follow-up. I would like to say here how important it is to look past all the meetings and documentation required toward "true improvement." It is very easy to spin your wheels by creating too many PI issues that can never be closed. It is far more effective to focus on those issues that [1] can cause severe harm, [2] have the potential to affect multiple patients, and [3] are reasonably correctable. True improvement often requires cooperation, consensus building, and collegiality. The sign of a truly effective leader of a trauma center is the person they can take a difficult issue that crosses many departments and care units, bring people together with a common cause, achieve a reachable goal, and document that they have made a difference.

Meetings

One of the core processes in any PI program is mandatory meetings. At a minimum there must be what the ACS describes as the mandatory attendance multi-disciplinary PI meeting. Many hospitals have more than one meeting, and often the site visit team will hold them to the attendance requirements the hospital has specified. But the mandatory attendance PI meeting should include the trauma medical director or the trauma program manager, all of the trauma faculty, liaisons, administrative personnel, and key unit personnel. Below is a sample agenda:

- Open discussion (10 minutes)
- Detailed review of mortalities with OFI (30 minutes)
- Synopsis of mortalities without OFI (10 minutes)
- Case review: complications, near misses, and significant morbidity (10 minutes)
- Operational issues (20 minutes)

    – Guidelines in development
    – Concerns from departments and units

- Review of PI and trauma center dashboard (5 minutes)

    – Open issues
    – Loop closure
    – Liaison and trauma surgeon attendance

- Final thoughts (5 minutes)

If the meeting is difficult to finish in less than 90 minutes a program may split the meeting into a peer-reviewed component (with only MDs and NP/PAs attending) and an operational meeting (open to all). Minutes and attendance must be recorded. As the program moves closer to its site review, 30 minutes may be added to discuss verification issues and problems.

These meetings are usually held monthly, and 50% attendance is required from the trauma medical director, the trauma surgeons, and the liaisons. Detailed minutes should be taken from these meetings in order to allow a site visitor to follow the path of the PI issue. Some states have restrictions on what can be documented in these meetings (for instance, Colorado and Kentucky), but it is incumbent upon the programs to develop a system by which they can prove that they are meeting all the key requirements of the PI program. This can include de-identifying PI records or aggregating PI issues such that they cannot be traced back to the individual patient.

The mandatory meeting at a minimum should include a review of all deaths, with special attention played to those deaths with opportunities for improvement, unanticipated mortalities. Some programs have separate system meetings where PI of EMS, aeromedical, and other parts of the trauma system are closely examined. In our own program, we devote a percentage of each mandatory meeting to system issues, and one of our PI techniques is that we try to aggregate individual PI issues into system projects that we then can devote our focus to a critical issue that effects many patients, instead of dividing our focus among a large number of small issues. Examples of system PI projects are:

- Massive transfusion protocol improvement
- Cervical spine clearance algorithm
- Creation of an ED trauma cart
- Multiple casualty incident planning
- Review of OR trauma cart supplies
- Blood utilization
- Improvement of hip fracture mortality
- Guidelines for communication on the trauma service

For our site visits, if a case was aggregated into a system OFI, we indicate the system project on the individual chart and provide the reviewers with the entire file on the system OFI including meeting minutes, problems encountered, deliverables, etc. We have received very positive feedback from our ACS and state site reviewers on this process.

Case Example

It is instructive to take a single PI case and demonstrate how it should pass through the system:

> A patient involved in a motor vehicle crash is transported by air to the trauma center, has the highest-level activation, suffers a severe head injury and spleen injuries as well as a severe pelvic fracture, and has an ICP bolt placed, external fixation of the pelvis, and laparotomy for splenectomy. The patient has a 10-day ICU course and then has a cardiac arrest on the acute care floor and cannot be resuscitated. Prior to the arrest, the patient was hemodynamically stable and had no laboratory abnormalities of any significance.

The trauma team will be aware of this patient and their death and may report the death themselves to the trauma program manager or medical director. Otherwise the trauma registrar should have a system to audit the outcomes of the trauma patients on the service on a daily basis and should be rapidly aware of the patients who died. What I will outline here is a common process of examination of the case like this.

The case will first be examined by the trauma program manager and/or the trauma PI coordinator. They will go into the chart or the registry entry and pull out the patient's initial vital signs on arrival of EMS, their initial vital signs on arrival in the emergency department, the conduct of the resuscitation and the timeliness of intervention, and whether protocols and guidelines were followed during this period of care. They will then assess the injuries found in the diagnostic phase and ensure documentation of all of these in the registry. The ICU care will then be examined with regard to ventilator pneumonia prevention, deep venous thrombosis prophylaxis, proper antibiotic use, administration of vaccines for the splenectomy, intracranial pressure, and cerebral perfusion pressure management (and timely management of any intracranial hypertension), mobilization of the patient when able, administration of nutrition, etc.

The events surrounding the patient's cardiac arrest would be thoroughly reviewed and documented including vital sign trends, oxygen saturation trends if available, administration of DVT prophylaxis, signs and symptoms of respiratory distress, physical therapy and occupational therapy documentation, and discussion with the nurses and nurse manager on the unit where the arrest occurred to see if any other information is available. Preferably the discussions with clinicians who interacted with the patient around the time of death would occur within 48 hours, preferably 24 hours after the event.

After this is documented in the PI record, the case will be discussed with the TMD to assess whether the death was anticipated and what further actions are needed. Let us say for the sake of example that the patient did not receive DVT prophylaxis for the 3 days prior to the cardiac arrest because the medication fell off the patient's medication administration list and was not renewed after it was stopped for orthopedic surgery. In addition, 2 hours prior to the patient's arrest, physical therapy (PT) documented that the patient became acutely short of breath upon getting out of bed for therapy. The patient was placed back in bed in the PT, and the patient felt more comfortable. No oxygen saturations were checked at this point, and vital signs were being obtained every 8 hours. With that data in mind, the patient appeared to be recovering and had no pending issues that would have led the team to believe the patient would not survive hospitalization.

Thus, the initial impression of the case would be that this was an unexpected death. In every unexpected death, it is vital that the PI program undertakes the most vigorous investigation. Unexpected deaths not only reveal process failures within the trauma center, but a site visit team will focus on unexpected deaths as examples of the power of the PI program to investigate themselves and make hard accountability decisions.

In rare instances, there may be no opportunity for improvement in an unexpected death. For instance, a patient is started at the appropriate time on the appropriate DVT prophylaxis, receives all the doses as ordered in the proper doses, and then dies of a pulmonary embolus. Assuming there are no other issues, based on the current care guidelines in the trauma center, there is no opportunity for improvement. However, the program should still look at the case very closely and ensure that all possible opportunities for improvement have been discussed. This outcome for an unexpected death should be rare.

In this case, there are several opportunities for improvement:

1. The patient's chemical prophylaxis was not given for several days after orthopedic surgery. This increased the risk of a DVT or PE.
2. The physical therapists concern over the patient's condition after getting the patient out of bed was not followed up.
3. Following this, the patient's general vital signs and their oxygen saturations specifically were not measured at reasonable intervals in a patient where a caregiver had expressed concern.

The initial findings above can pass through several processes depending on the center. In many centers, these findings would be discussed between the TPM and TMD who would decide on the next steps. In others, a PI coordinator would discuss this with the program manager or medical director, and the case would be presented at a working PI meeting. (*Many programs have "working PI meetings" in addition to their mandatory attendance multidisciplinary PI meeting. The purpose of this smaller meeting, which often only includes the PI coordinator, and PI medical director, or the TPM and TMD, or some other combination, is to attack problems more rapidly than would be possible if all cases had to wait for discussion at the larger MDPI meeting*).

The initial case review and analysis have been completed, OFIs have been identified, and the initial discussion has occurred between the key players in the trauma PI process. At this point there are several directions that this could go:

- In less than mature programs, the case will be presented at the multidisciplinary performance improvement meeting with the findings up to this point, and the entire group would be asked to comment and suggest corrective actions.

This is done in less than mature programs because they need to have buy-in from all involved parties before moving forward, and the MDPI meeting is the best way to do that.

- However, in most mature PI programs, the TPM and TMD or their designate would begin to construct corrective actions and then bring in people from the areas involved to work out the actual processes for improvement. Waiting for the MDPI meeting to discuss the case would be a waste of time when these system issues may harm another patient. A mature program should be able to define and initiate corrective actions in a case such as this rapidly.

The medication issue in this case concerns the DVT prophylaxis falling off the patient's medications after the orthopedic surgery. This can be addressed in several ways:

- If there is an electronic medical record that is adaptable, the program can work with the local computing resources to add a prompt or best practice alert to any patients' chart when they meet criteria for high risk for DVT such that the clinician is prompted to either start chemical prophylaxis or type in an explanation as to why it has not been started if the program identifies the patient is not receiving prophylaxis. Such a best practice alert in this case would most likely have warned the provider that the medication had fallen off the patient's administration list and it would've been added back in. However, many electronic medical records are not this adaptable, and other solutions need to be worked out.
- The program can initiate standard work for the postoperative trauma patient. This can include a checklist that is documented and retained in the record or some other processes. This standard work can be disseminated to all clinicians and monitored for compliance. In our program we created practice guidelines 25 years ago [2] and update them twice a year since then. These guidelines are distributed to all nurses and physicians, nurse practitioners, physician assistants that work with our patients, as well as pharmacists. These guidelines are constantly updated in an

iPhone/Google Play application [3] that is free to anyone who would like to use it. All of our residents, medical students, nurses, NP/PAs, and physicians can consult our guidelines at any time. In this case our guidelines are fairly clear that a patient with these injuries with a stable hematocrit would have chemical prophylaxis restarted with a delay of no more than 24 hours. But no guideline mandates the actual physical task of placing the appropriate orders. And when clinicians get busy, critical tasks can be forgotten, especially on evenings where patients come back from the operating room and there are multiple admissions and critical ICU patients. This is why it is vital to involve the nursing staff in the maintenance of high-quality care. In this case our process would be to bring together the nursing leadership in the units where we practice to discuss how we can use checklists to ensure that delays will be eliminated. In fact, this is the corrective action we have taken in similar cases on several occasions at my institution.

The corrective action for the second issue is more complicated. In this case physical therapist documented that they felt the patient had become more dyspneic after an exercise session and wanted this followed up. It can often be difficult to find out how this information was transferred after the fact. We feel that simply writing these findings in the chart is not sufficient if the clinician is truly worried about a change in patient condition. With the explosion of data in the electronic medical record, it would be almost impossible to ensure that every note written by every clinician would be read on every patient every day; thus, another system has to be put in place.

The system needs to stress that all the clinicians taking care of the trauma patient work as a team. This includes everyone from housekeeping, to nutrition services, to the surgeon in charge. All members of the team need to feel empowered to bring to the highest levels any serious concern about the patient's condition. We stress this to all our clinicians. It can be difficult especially after unexpected death to truly discern how much worry there was about the change in patient's condition. After clinicians find out that the patient had an unexpected death, past observations that may have warned the staff can be inflated in retrospect. That is why it is vital to stress to people to bring these concerns to the proper people rapidly so that no information is lost with time. As you can see, this is a tougher corrective action and requires less concrete actions on the part of the trauma program. What would be expected from the site reviewer who is looking at a chart like this would be that there was discussion, that the PI program took the physical therapist concerns seriously and interface with the physical therapists to figure out a system by which they could report changes in patient condition to the proper people rapidly, and that these reports would be given adequate weight.

The third issue is also complex. When there is an unexpected death, people will go back and look at what was done and give small "errors" greater weight in the face of the known outcome. In this case, the program should carefully look back at the situation as it presented itself around the time when the physical therapist determined that there had been a change in patient condition. If they could not determine that there was any examination of the patient by the nursing staff for a period of time greater than that which was ordered, then it would be an opportunity for improvement that needs to be brought up and closed with the nursing staff. However, in many of these cases, hindsight is 20/20, and people will say that we should have obtained more data, measured oxygen saturations more frequently, etc. What is expected in the loop closure for these types of issues is that they are thoroughly discussed, and all members of the team are given a chance to comment and are given a chance to propose solutions, and that if concrete solutions can be made to prevent this from happening to another patient in the future that those solutions are implemented and properly documented.

References

1. Committee on Trauma, American College of Surgeons. Resource for optimal care of the injured patient. 2014. https://www.facs.org/-/media/files/quality-programs/trauma/vrc-resources/resources-for-optimal-care.ashx?la=en.
2. Young JS. Trauma manual. 2019. https://www.medicalcenter.virginia.edu/intranet/trauma-center/trauma-manual-spring-2019.
3. Young S. UVa Trauma, Version 1.2.5, Apple App Store and Google Play.

Chapter 13
The Performance Improvement Process

Tier 1: TPM and TMD

The TPM and TMD are key players in an effective PI program. Even if your program uses a PI coordinator and associate medical director in charge of PI, the TPM and TMD will often be called upon for difficult issues and for loop closure that involves specialties or other hospital departments. While it is expected under normal circumstances for the PI staff to work with the unit managers and liaisons to correct problems, it is frequent that the TPM will often have to intercede in complex nursing and administrative issues, and the TMD will often have to work on complex physician and NP/PA issues.

This is one of the reasons why novices should not be in these roles. To have an effective, efficient trauma center, relationships must be strong among key players. If the trauma center leadership acts arrogantly or in a dictatorial fashion, they will likely not be in those positions for very long, and the trauma center may be set back a considerable amount by that type of leadership, since relationships will need to be rebuilt by the replacements.

© Springer Nature Switzerland AG 2020
J. S. Young, *Trauma Centers*,
https://doi.org/10.1007/978-3-030-34607-2_13

These are good rules of thumb:

1. Always put the patient's best interests first. That should be the basis of any discussion.
2. When there is no clear evidence that one path is better than the other, try to reach an agreement on a reasonable path. If there is no clear scientific standard, you must be willing to compromise.
3. On critical issues where a patient's life was, or may be, put in danger, and where the standard of care is clear, do not compromise, especially when the person is persisting in putting their needs above the needs of the patient.
4. Don't be out on a ledge. If you are having trouble with a loop closure, gather data (to make sure you are on the correct side of the truth), gather allies, and if necessary, escalate to higher authorities.

Tier 2: The Multidisciplinary Performance Improvement (MDPI) Meeting

This meeting is done by different names in different institutions. But, basically, this is the meeting that is mandated by the American College of Surgeons and most states where the trauma director, trauma surgeons, specialty liaisons, and representatives of key departments need to discuss performance improvement. After the TPM and TMD have formed a corrective action plan and done some preliminary discussions on a case, it can now be presented at MDPI for discussion with other key contributors of the trauma program. Often at the MDPI meeting, people will make helpful suggestions and may discuss ways that they can help facilitate solutions. Also there can be contentious discussions at these meetings where specialty surgeons or departments feel the corrective action plan is placing undue burden on them. Therefore, this is where the trauma medical director is really put to the test by supervising difficult conversations and overcoming resistance in creating a safer and more effective trauma center.

The MDPI meeting is usually monthly but can be less frequent at less busy programs, although monthly meetings are the norm. Most mature programs have another meeting every month or every week where a smaller group discusses new PI cases and discusses the progress on old ones. This intermediate meeting is not mandated by the American College of Surgeons or by any states that I'm aware of but is often extremely useful in moving PI issues along. If every PI issue waits for the mandatory monthly meeting, then progress often has to wait several weeks, and a weekly meeting allows things to move quicker. The PI meeting should have an agenda that is distributed to all attendees sufficiently ahead of time. If the agenda contains patient information, it should be distributed in a secure manner without any possibility of forwarding. In addition, it is often optimal for the PI meeting to be guided by slides; the usual process is introduction, review of agenda and past minutes of meetings, discussion of mortalities and opportunities for improvement, and discussion of cases where loop closure is still pending. In these cases, it is important to talk about the progress and overcome obstacles. There should also be an open part of the session for people to bring up problems that they have seen in patient care. Finally most programs including my own present a dashboard to the committee. This dashboard is usually updated quarterly and shows patient outcomes, transfers from outside hospitals, mortality rates for different ISS classes, and a variety of other information. This dashboard is not mandated by regulatory agencies that I'm aware of, but it is a good way to keep the key members of the program informed of how the year is going.

Tier 3:   In this tier, the cases have been reviewed by the TPM, the TMD, and the PI committee, but further action is needed that will involve the hospital administration or the clinical departments. The TPM and TMD usually interact with either the hospital quality program, the executive suite, or the leadership of the departments to allocate a portion of the corrective action plan to them. This type of PI action can often create problems. Hospital departmental PI processes usually move much slower than the trauma programs, so those cases that are sent to these entities for action often encounter significant delays in closure. I've seen many instances where the trauma program has done an outstanding job in laying out the corrective action plan for hospital administration or a clinical department, and then there is no response for months despite frequent inquiries. In fact this is really quite common. This is why I often recommend that some key member of the trauma program (either the TPM, the TMD, or the PI coordinator) interact regularly with the hospital quality program and should attend meetings where the performance of various centers in the medical center is discussed.

Opportunities for improvement are the key component of performance improvement. These are issues in the case that may or may not have negatively affected the outcome but which were suboptimal. One of the most difficult things to assess as a site reviewer is the diligence by which the program identifies opportunities for improvement. Mature trauma programs will often triage opportunities according to the potential harm to the patient or the chance of recurrence. This is because mature programs have dealt with complex issues before and fix them effectively. In an immature program, the site reviewer may be concerned if they see that opportunities for improvement that are identified are not corrected. Regardless, any opportunity for improvement that harms the patient whether it appears to be uncommon or whether it is something that touches every trauma patient or only a few should undergo the cycle of analysis, corrective action, and loop closure.

Every trauma program needs to triage its opportunities for improvement. There are some issues that must be dealt with in an "emergent" basis, for example, lack of blood availability in an emergency situation, drug shortages for essential medications, critical staffing issues, etc. Then there are issues that can go through the routine PI process that have been described including TPM/PI coordinator evaluation, discussion with the

TMD, creation of corrective action plans, presentation of the multidisciplinary PI meeting, and loop closure. Our program categorizes certain opportunities for improvement as "projects." We outlined those projects in a previous chapter. Opportunities for improvement are put in this category if correction will require a wide-ranging multidisciplinary effort, often involving administration, budgeting, and coordination among multiple units and services. We placed these issues in this category also because trying to solve these problems piecemeal will often be ineffective. Therefore, we choose several of these "projects" every year and devote an allocated amount of PI effort to them. During our site visit, we present to the team that these opportunities for improvement are "non-case based," meaning that we would prefer that they not go back to the individual cases but look at the overall PI effort and loop closure. I will explain better in the site visit section how to demonstrate these PI efforts to site visit team.

The following are lists of typical opportunities for improvement with subcategories of criticality:

- Missed injury

  - Missed orthopedic injury
  - Missed laceration
  - Lack of follow-up of known neurologic injury
  - Missed spine injuries

- Significant adverse event or complication

  - Pneumonia
  - Urinary tract infection
  - Pressure ulcer
  - Fall
  - Medication error
  - Wound infection
  - Intra-abdominal abscess
  - Delay in treatment
  - Failure to rescue
  - Cardiac arrest
  - Unexpected return to the O
  - Unexpected extubation

- Inefficiency and delay
  - Delay in radiology reads
  - Incorrect initial radiology interpretation
  - Delay in CT scan availability
  - Delay in operating room availability
  - Delay in blood product availability
  - Delay in specialist consultation
  - Delay in attending involvement

There are many materials available to outline the PI efforts that would address these opportunities for improvement. I refer the reader to the TOPIC course created by the Society of Trauma Nurses and the optimal trauma care course created jointly by the ACS Committee on Trauma and Society of Trauma Nurses (https://www.traumanurses.org/optimal) [1].

After you have identified opportunities for improvement, the next step is to discuss the opportunities/event with the relevant parties. Remember that up to this point, little frontline input has been acquired. Even with outstanding documentation, you will miss subtleties in the case and potentially chase down an insignificant opportunity for improvement or miss a significant one.

The discussion of a significant opportunity for improvement parallels the process for a root cause analysis. This involves creating a timeline of the events, identifying the key clinicians involved in the care, and either contacting them directly or scheduling a meeting where everyone could sit in the same room and discuss the case. In many busy trauma programs, the PI coordinator will take the case and speak to a group of individuals separately since, as we all know, trying to set up a meeting with a dozen busy clinicians can delay action for a significant period of time.

Once the timeline is created, the trauma program manager/trauma medical director/PI coordinator and occasionally the specialty liaison will go over the timeline to decide at what points opportunities exist. Many opportunities for improvement can entail multiple problems. It is rare that a significant adverse outcome is the result of a single decision or action. Often a single action is followed by another suboptimal action that then leads the patient down an unrecoverable path. Thus, the team should not stop after finding a single opportunity but should go through the entire timeline to ensure that they are identifying everything that might be relevant to future patient care.

There is a difference of opinion on the extent of documentation of this investigation. I believe at the very least the PI record should include who is contacted, the substance of the conversation, and whether that conversation led down different paths or led to a corrective action which could led to closure. Remember that these discussions are outside of the multidisciplinary PI venue. These discussions often will go on primarily within the trauma program, with input from clinicians and specialists. Many opportunities for improvement can be closed with simple discussion as long as there is documentation that the discussion took place and that no further action was needed. As we will discuss in the site visit chapters, there are certainly events that do not require anything more than a simple investigation and closure. However, the program must be wary of using this type of closure frequently. Site visitors will be suspicious if events that may have contributed to adverse outcomes are closed without corrective action and loop closure. This does not mean you can never do it. It just means that you should not always do it.

Reference

1. Society of Trauma Nurses. Optimal trauma center organization & management course. 2019. https://www.traumanurses.org/optimal. Accessed 24 Sept 2019

Chapter 14
Mortality Review and the Multidisciplinary Performance Improvement Meeting

After you've analyzed an opportunity for improvement and have had some preliminary discussions, you need to take the issue through the rest of the PI process. The TOPIC course [1] teaches four levels of case review. Level I is the primary review which we have already talked about that includes the identification of the event, the confirmation of the event, immediate feedback from frontline caregivers, and initial discussion among the trauma program leadership. Many OFIs and cases can be closed at this level if it is determined by the program leadership that no further review is necessary. Again, as I said earlier, a PI program needs to be implemented carefully so that significant issues that are persistent in the care of the injured patient can be investigated thoroughly. But there is a misunderstanding often on the part of trauma centers during site visits that everything must undergo complete review.

In the TOPIC rubric, the next level of review involves evaluation of the medical record and the development of timeline by the trauma medical director or trauma program manager. Many cases can be closed at this level as well. Cases that go for secondary review may be referred to the multidisciplinary committee, a trauma or departmental morbidity and mortality conferences, or a trauma center system committee if not integrated into the MDPI committee. The next level involves review at a formal committee. These could be the multidisciplinary peer-reviewed committee, another PI committee, regional trauma committees, prehospital quality committees, or hospital quality and patient safety conferences. The final level of review usually involves external peer review and review by the hospital quality committee. These often involve sentinel events. Please enroll in the TOPIC course for more information as I've given a very cursory review of the process that they recommend.

While my trauma center does not formally use these levels of review, the levels of review that I described are fairly intuitive. What we will discuss here is preparing cases for your multidisciplinary PI committee, how the discussion should be conducted, and how the events should be recorded.

The trauma center leadership (trauma program manager, trauma program medical director, trauma PI coordinator, and possibly the trauma registrar) reviews the cases that will be presented at the multidisciplinary committee and ensures that committee members can follow the clinical timeline of the patient. If an action plan is to be presented that involves another department or unit, it is critical that the program leadership discuss this with those entities before assigning an action plan in front of the entire committee. This will avoid tension and conflict at the committee which is often detrimental to the performance improvement process. If slides are going to detail deficiencies on the part of a unit, department, or specialty, these should be reviewed with those entities prior to the meeting so that you may obtain their input. I want to stress that it does not mean that these issues are not discussed. *Surprising clinicians and administrators with detailed information about suboptimal performance in front of a large group of peers is not an effective way to conduct performance improvement.* Trauma centers that do things this way often have constant conflict between specialties, the trauma service, OR, ED, and other areas. It is the special quality of effective trauma center leadership to know how to gain consensus and performance improvement through collaboration, communication, and a willingness to see both sides of any issue. But it is the trauma medical director's job to ensure trauma care continually improves. There will often be instances where certain entities will be complacent and happy with the current state of their performance. After discussing issues with them and hearing their side of the story, if they still will not work toward improving quality and patient safety, then the committee can be used as a vehicle to place peer pressure upon them for compliance and improvement.

We will often start with a period of appreciative inquiry where we ask the group if they would like to share any events that made them particularly proud to work at the trauma center (and hopefully there will be one or two) and move into case review. As I stated previously, the case review should include a general description of the patient, their care before arriving at the trauma center, their care in the emergency department, their initial diagnostic work-up, their initial procedures and operations, and a summary of their clinical course and their outcomes. In a case presentation template, you should include the demographic data including injury severity score and probability of survival. We feel this provides a committee member with information about whether the outcome, if it was a poor outcome, was anticipated based on a high injury severity and/or a low probability of survival. Then the case should include a timeline of events. This could be in a chart or in a bullet-pointed list. Then you should list the opportunities for improvement that have been identified or if none have been identified the recommendation to close the case. If you do recommend closure, the committee should be queried as to whether there are any questions or any concerns, and they should be recorded. It is vital during your site visit that you demonstrate that cases that are closed without action were reviewed by more than one person and that the decision to close the case was logical.

For those cases where OFIs have been identified, the program should list the issue, some of their analysis, and the recommendations for corrective action. The committee should discuss these recommendations and determine how the center will know that the loop has been closed. In many cases, loop closure involves ongoing audit of performance. This is completely acceptable, especially for rare events without evidence of significant harm. A problem with some PI programs is when many issues are triaged to ongoing audit. In many of these cases, when the site visit team asked for evidence of an ongoing audit none is available. Thus, "ongoing audit" is used as a way to avoid addressing the problem by making it appear that the corrective action was implemented, but you have no idea whether the new process is being followed.

It is also vital that the program keeps track of all the OFIs that have been identified, and what stage of review these issues are currently at (for instance, TPM review, TMD review, liaison review, hospital quality committee review, or specialty department review). This log should also include the responsible person and the product that is required for loop closure (for instance, a letter from a liaison, a new guideline, a new protocol for patient care unit, etc.). We integrate all of these things into one database so that if a letter, guideline, protocol, or any other product is created for the purpose of loop closure of an OFI, we have a link to this in our log so that it could rapidly be reviewed by the PI program or site visit team. While many programs use many different methods to corral their PI activities, you have to ask yourself "if I have to demonstrate that we addressed this issue, how could I do it?" Remember that site visits often occur every 3 years and you may be required to demonstrate your performance improvement process in a case that is 10–12 months old or longer. I reviewed programs where I've seen cases that had corrective action plans that were open for several years. This is not necessarily a deficiency, but the program has to have a good reason why they were unable to close out this issue.

Disposition

There are a variety of ways to dispose off PI issues and we have already discussed several of them. To reiterate, an issue can be closed at the TPM level, at the TMD level, at the MDPI level, or at the hospital quality level. Very few issues make it all the way to the hospital quality level as, short of sentinal events, the hospital administration usually expects the programs to be able to correct most OFI's.

There are several processes to close an OFI. First is documentation of closure at a lower level. What a site reviewer will expect, and what you should expect from your own program, are issues that are closed without significant discussion or analysis are for the most part trivial or issues where little harm came to the patient, and the potential for future harm is very low. For the former, I have seen OFIs for team conduct in the resuscitation bay. This includes members of the team sniping and other members of the team raising their voice or being derogatory. While I am not implying that these are always trivial, they can be handled locally and don't usually represent a systemic problem within the trauma center. However, even with issues such as this if they are recurrent and if they are interfering with the effectiveness of the team, then they would need to be elevated. For the latter, these issues represent problems where closure is simply not possible in our current day and age. These would include some socioeconomic issues, issues around certain types of needle injuries, or even issues revolving around the refusal of organ donation for families. My point here is that to track down issues of that type would very likely require tremendous amounts of effort and would require input from more than just a trauma center or the hospital, and thus it would be acceptable to say that these issues will be closed pending local action.

For other issues that are closed at either the MDPI level or the TMD/TPM level, documentation of the preliminary analysis along with the relation of the opportunity to the ideal state and the necessary countermeasures should be included. These are most commonly simple laboratory or departmental issues that are fixed by the TPM or TMD by discussing and implementing appropriate countermeasures. Documentation of these discussions, the plan of action, and monitoring for further problems should be included. I will try to talk about examples of this in the case studies.

For OFIs that are more complex and involve changes in practice, guideline development, clinician performance issues, or large projects meant to improve the outcomes for populations of patients, the documentation should be more rigorous. This would include documentation of analysis and decision-making outside of the committee structure, documentation of meetings with individuals necessary to implement practice change, and summarizing meetings where guidelines were discussed and developed. You should also document the processes for implementation of guidelines, and monitoring of outcomes. In general, these issues are extremely complex, and your average trauma program cannot have more than two or three of these per year. But issues such as this where it is obvious that the trauma program has spent a great deal of time and effort to improve a process that will have a positive impact on a large number of patients are extremely impressive not only to your administration but to the site visit team. The program should consider turning these projects into publications (after institutional review board approval) so other centers can learn how they carried out a complex process improvement project and demonstrated a positive effect on outcomes.

Monitoring

Monitoring should be used either to assess the effectiveness of the corrective action plan or to determine whether an OFI is occurring with sufficient frequency to warrant more intense investigation. Not every OFI needs a full investigation, and often there are "one-off" incidents where the replication of the problem is unlikely. However, if such an incident led to an extremely adverse outcome, it is important for the program to monitor for recurrence.

For what we call "issue auditing," the program should develop a simple method for monitoring the occurrence of an adverse event or recurrence of a process issue. The program should set the defined interval for the auditing so that they can demonstrate to the site visit team that they looked at the problem closely for a fixed period of time and concluded that it was fixed and did not require further intervention. There are some things that may require open-ended auditing, but they should be rare because if the program states that they are auditing something indefinitely, then they may be required to produce documentation to show that they are continuing to gather data.

Brent James at Intermountain Healthcare says that your auditing process should not be complicated. The more time you spend creating a complicated monitoring process, the less time you're actually looking at the problem. Monitoring tools could be as simple as a sheet of paper with checkboxes or a process by which clinicians can email someone in the trauma program every time there is a deviation. The latter process is a little bit less rigorous in that all you are looking for is when people deviate from the process and not how many times they are adhering to it.

In summary, the program should choose carefully what processes to audit. The audits should have a lifespan, and the results of the audits should be easily accessible to the program and to site visitors.

Trigger for Further Action

The program also needs to be mindful that not all problems are fixed the first time. This can become apparent if a major clinical care issue recurs, clinicians inform the program that a problem is not been fixed, or auditing reveals that the corrective action plan didn't succeed. It is truly the sign of a mature program to look back at corrective actions and adjust them based on their performance. Demonstrating this to administration and a site visit team can make the program look very good. It seems obvious that you should always make certain that corrective actions work, but you would be surprised the number of times that a corrective action is created on paper, distributed, and then never looked at again until a similar problem rears its head.

The process for redirecting a corrective action is the same as the initial process. Look at the problem, analyze it carefully, look closely at the reasons for failure, create countermeasures, and then audit the new process.

One problem many programs encounter is where to place this type of information in the performance improvement records. It is very difficult to tie a complex corrective action plan that crosses populations and service lines back to a single patient. In fact I would advise you not to link these types of things directly to a single patient, even though a single patient may have instigated the process. It is far more effective to create a separate project or folder that encompasses the problem, its corrective action, and monitoring. Every program should have several folders like this where major clinical and system issues are constantly evaluated for performance. In our own program, we have folders such as this for rapid evacuation of mass lesions in the head, massive transfusion protocol performance, safe interhospital transfer, etc. Moreover, the folder should be kept updated and celebrated for success. As we will discuss in the site visit section, many visitors will expect PI issues to be intimately tied back to individual patients. One way that we do this is to assign OFIs to system folders and, in the actual patient PI record, indicate that the problem has been triaged into a system project. Then when the visitors look at the chart, they will say "where is the loop closure on this?" And we can present them with documentation of how that incident or several similar incidents led to a large PI effort that was effective.

Corrective Actions

Abstract: Here we describe the most common corrective actions used in the performance improvement process. We also detail the problems with each, and what the site visit team will expect when they examine these corrective actions.

Education

"Education" is often the most common corrective action taken by PI programs (other than "no PI issue identified"). It is also a red flag to site reviewers. It is simple to document "education" as a corrective action, but it is extremely difficult to prove that it effectively addressed the relevant issue. Here is an example:

A 49-year-old woman was admitted to the trauma center following an automobile crash. Initial prehospital report indicated the patient was awake but confused and exhibited a closed left femur fracture and bruising along the left chest. Vital signs on the first report were 120/78, pulse 90, with normal oxygen saturations. Five minutes prior to arrival, the crew radios that the patient's blood pressure has dropped to 70/40 and pulse increased to 120. The report is acknowledged by the emergency medicine attending. No trauma activation is called, and the patient arrives in extremis. The trauma team is not present, and an activation is called 10 minutes after arrival. When the team arrives, they encounter a dismal situation with an unstable patient. They proceed through normal tasks, intubate the patient, and start transfusing blood. The FAST is positive, and the patient is taken to the OR where she undergoes splenectomy. The patient has a rocky postoperative course with acute kidney injury and pneumonia but is discharged to rehabilitation.

The trauma program clearly identifies the undertriage based on the final prehospital report. Their corrective action is "education of the emergency medicine attending."

The corrective action in this case may seem reasonable at first glance; however when you look deeper, it can reveal a very superficial review. A mature program would make certain that this attending had not been guilty of other undertriaging other patients. They would ensure that if an activation was not initiated, other ED personnel would feel empowered to correct the error. Meaning that when this patient arrives, providers in the emergency department would know this patient met trauma activation criteria and there was a solid process for rapidly activating the trauma team. The program should also ask why was there a delay? Was it because clinicians felt intimidated? Was the patient not evaluated immediately on arrival?

Next, in a case like this, a thorough reviewer would ask "what's your incidence of these types of events?" and "how many patients are upgraded after arrival in the ED?" These questions could reveal a system that is not adequate with regard to assessing prehospital information accurately or a reluctance to activate the trauma team (which is a more serious issue). Reviewers know that this should have been a highest level activation and need to make certain the EM physicians are not intimidated by surgeons to see patients before activating the team. I have seen in centers where the trauma surgeon is not in house at night, there may be an unwritten understanding with the ED not to call alerts unless absolutely necessary in order to avoid overtriage.

As you can see, a program needs to be careful in the extensive use of education as a corrective action. It is certainly appropriate in "one-off" instances where the system runs smoothly and someone just did something wrong. But repeated use of this action would indicate an immature PI program.

Internal Education Program

The internal education program (IEP) was a concept developed by the ACS to encourage centers to use more directed learning techniques. The goal was to have the PI program use wide-reaching educational offerings to inform many members of the trauma center team of aberrancies, new protocols, new evidence from the literature, etc. Using a broad-ranging educational tool to address an opportunity for improvement is actually viewed favorably. That is because this implies that the PI staff looked deeply into the problem, spent time formulating an educational plan, and created and distributed that plan. Also there is evidence that the education went out, and often these tools are rolled into the hospital internal education program so there is often documentation that the offering was read and questions were answered to demonstrate understanding of the issue. Many programs use the IEP extensively to inform all staff of errors and corrections, new guidelines, and good saves. Educational corrective actions that are carried out using an IEP often demonstrate an effective PI program.

Guideline

Guidelines can be the most difficult corrective action to carry out. This is due to the fact that many hospitals have extensive rules for publishing guidelines (committee review, retirement or renewal after 2–3 years, etc.). It is unfortunate that these restrictions on guideline creation often inhibit their use since they can be very effective.

In our program, we have published a guideline manual yearly since 1994 [1]. In the past 5 years, the published manual has been converted into a smartphone application [2] that all residents and staff download to have at their fingertips. Serious issues or new evidence lead to off-cycle revisions if they are significant.

Relevant and well thought out guidelines tend to have the most beneficial effect on suboptimal care. Brent James from Intermountain Healthcare taught that guidelines are merely a tool to measure variation. Without guidelines, we have chaos and individual "ego-based" medicine. If you don't have something to measure your current decisions against, then you have no logical way to correct problems and instigate change.

You should not strive for perfection in guideline creation. Only 20–30% of the care we deliver is supported by the highest level evidence; thus, experience and judgment will play a role in almost every clinical decision. However, I like to teach that there is no reason to have to cogitate on 100% of the things that you do in medicine. Do you have to think about whether you should check a complete blood count every morning for each patient, or can you sit down and decide that you will order CBCs until you have 2 days where the values are stable? Another teaching point is that guidelines are merely a way to write experience down for the inexperienced. Every guideline should be vetted with expert, experienced clinicians, and their honest logical concerns should be given weight.

Creation of Guidelines

Guidelines often grow out of PI problems. An example is what method should be used to clear the spine of an unconscious patient. As experienced traumatologists know, this is a difficult subject that is constantly changing in the literature. Our process for the creation of this guideline was first to examine the latest evidence. Google Scholar can be a good source, and the Journal of Trauma and the Eastern Association for the Surgery of Trauma (EAST) guidelines are also excellent sources. EAST guidelines are created by groups of trauma surgeons with specific rules for evaluation of evidence. When reading any of these practice guidelines, it is important that you go back and read the cited key literature. Having been a part of these guideline committees, I have seen individual preferences of the chair, and biased reviews of publication leads to guidelines that tend to lean in one direction or another, rather than completely representing an unbiased review. This is only natural since the committee members have a great deal of clinical experience, and there are few randomized prospective trials in trauma surgery, so opinion will need to be a part of the process.

For this example, our PI team was informed of a pressure ulcer in a critically injured trauma patient where the cervical collar had rubbed against the patient's occiput. The patient's cervical spine CT was negative, but our protocol at that time stated that if the patient was not awake enough to tell us they had no cervical pain, an MRI was required to remove the cervical collar. This protocol grew out of the data indicating (at that time) that up to 5% of cervical spine injuries are ligamentous, and they will not be detected on CT. Though the chance of a significant injury was very low with a negative CT, at that time, there was a difference of opinion in the country regarding this process, and we erred on the side of caution.

After this pressure ulcer was discovered, we re-evaluated the literature and brought in the orthopedic and neurosurgical spine specialists who help with standardizing spine care. There was a clear disagreement between the specialists; one said that a clean dedicated spine CT was sufficient (which was consistent with the majority of recent spine literature), and the other still felt the unconscious patient required a clean MRI for clearance. The trauma program went into the literature and consensus statements and re-presented the general national consensus to both specialists and brought in one other spine surgeon from each department. After about 4 weeks, we created a guideline that incorporated a completely negative spine CT as sufficient for clearance; however, any abnormality on the CT required an MRI.

This brings up another important concept in trauma center management, what if someone you ask for an opinion is an outlier? They disagree with the consensus, and you sense they will actively undermine the guideline if pushed through. If you believe this physician is sincere, can present their thoughts logically, and that they can compromise to some extent, their concerns should be incorporated into your guideline to some extent. This is why it is important to choose the experts in your institution and not just any specialist who will answer your email. If this person is respected and is putting the patient first (and not their ego), then it is a tactical error to ignore them completely. This creates tension and conflict that could spread to that entire department and creates an enemy who could take an active role in undermining the care the program wishes to deliver. Also, almost everything in medicine is an educated guess (some more educated than others) so you can never be certain that this specialist is completely wrong, but you do not need to have a guideline held hostage by one physician. If this physician will not reasonably compromise, then you may need to escalate to a division chief or chair for their opinion. That way if the superior contradicts the specialist, then the blame for that can be placed on someone other than the trauma program. In this case, one specialist felt that the CT was sufficient and that some injuries on CT that were minor could be ignored, and the other wanted MRI in all cases but agreed that a completely normal spine CT was sufficient. Thus, the compromise was that the CT must be completely negative to remove the collar. Any traumatic abnormality required MRI. The guideline was put in place, and soon our time to collar removal in ICU patients dropped by 50%, and our MRI utilization in these patients dropped by 40%.

Distribution

Many programs struggle with how to disseminate new and existing guidelines. As I stated previously, we have a system that includes smartphone applications that can be updated, immediately if necessary. This tool is not available to most programs, and other solutions need to be found.

I have seen many tools and here are a few. First, in many programs, the guideline is discussed at their MDPI meeting, and the liaisons and surgeons are tasked with disseminating the guideline. This is usually a suboptimal process in that each liaison and committee member will have a different method for spread (conversation, email, poster, etc.), and each will have different efficacy. It is not surprising that in many programs, discussion at MDPI does not adequately spread new guidelines. Another method is a "newsletter" distributed by the program at set intervals. This provides documentation of the dissemination but again may not be opened and read. This loop can be closed by incorporating the newsletter (or other type of educational program) into the hospital's learning management system. In that scenario, there is documentation that the information was read (or at least opened) and test questions can be incorporated to better assess comprehension. This along with discussion at MDPI is a common effective method.

A effective tool is a PI coordinator or clinical nurse specialist who attends rounds regularly to audit and insure that the guideline is known and is being followed. This is probably the best method in that the program can know that the issue is being addressed on rounds and that the new guideline is being used.

Auditing

Auditing of guideline use can be difficult. Clinical teams have enough to do on rounds and usually are not happy about recording whether a guideline is used or if there is deviation and why. As stated above, a physical presence on rounds is perhaps the best method, but not all decisions are made on rounds.

I recommend looking at the reason you created the guideline in the first place. If it was a reaction to an adverse event, measure the new rate of the adverse event. In the example above, pressure ulcer cases are recorded by the hospital wound care team and are reported through our safety report system. If a pressure ulcer occurs on a trauma patient, the team may report it to the PI coordinator, but more often the hospital will report the event to the trauma program for comment. This allows us to determine whether the event was related to the guideline (e.g., the ulcer may have occurred in a patient with an unstable spine; thus, the guideline was not relevant) and allows us to count the rate of the event and report it through the program. Success can also be celebrated through MDPI and email.

Clinical Staff Action

In rare instances, clinical staff action may need to be taken. This is a difficult step in the PI process because this may involve terminating someone's employment. A program that uses this method frequently will not be successful in that it demonstrates there simply is not enthusiasm and support for a trauma center if multiple clinicians will simply not follow the plan. Obviously, this should not be used for trivial matters, but issues where the patient's life may have been put at risk or where the clinician appeared to be negligent.

In many hospitals, removing privileges for a certain type of care requires clinical staff committee action. For instance, the TMD by themselves often cannot remove the privileges for trauma care. This may seem to be in conflict with the trauma center criteria that state the TMD must have the authority to remove someone from the trauma panel, but realistically unless the TMD is a division chief or chair, they simply do not possess this authority. What site visitors will look for is not whether the TMD had the individual authority to remove someone, but whether the hospital followed the recommendations of the TMD. If those recommendations are ignored and a dangerous clinician is still allowed to care for injured patients, then this will be a critical deficiency. Thus, policing the conduct of the physicians is both a trauma program and hospital responsibility.

Some examples for clinical staff action include not responding to a request for an emergency consult when unencumbered by other clinical duties, substance abuse while on call, consistently unable to respond to the highest level activation. If after counseling and sufficient warnings, the clinician is repeatedly carrying out care that is in conflict with routine trauma center guidelines (e.g., repeatedly not obtaining abdominal cross-sectional imaging for clear and indisputable indications) then the program may initiate a clinical staff action through the hospital.

References

1. Society of Trauma Nurses. Trauma outcomes and performance improvement course. Lexington; 2015.
2. Young S. UVa Trauma, Version 1.2.5, Apple App Store and Google Play.

Chapter 15
Benchmarking and Optimization

Benchmarking Systems

There are many outcomes that can be benchmarked (length of stay, cost, reimbursement, various complication, mortality rate, etc.). In order to properly compare centers, risk adjustment is critical. We will not go into all the vagaries of risk adjustment but will explain some of the principles.

As an example, we will examine benchmarking of mortality rate. To compare mortality rates between or within medical centers, the first step is to determine the individual's risk of mortality or calculate the risk of mortality for a group of patients with similar characteristics. The TRISS system (also known as the probability of survival) used in trauma [1] uses the Revised Trauma Score [2] and the Injury Severity Score [3] to calculate probability of survival (POS) [4] for each patient. These scores are entered into an equation developed through logistic regression of large populations of trauma patients generating a number for POS. This website allows you to calculate the probability of survival by entering the scores for injuries in individual organ systems (the ISS), the age, mechanism of injury, initial blood pressure, respiratory rate, and Glasgow Coma

© Springer Nature Switzerland AG 2020   177
J. S. Young, *Trauma Centers*,
https://doi.org/10.1007/978-3-030-34607-2_15

Scale (http://www.trauma.org/archive/scores/triss.html). For instance, a patient with a closed femur fracture, grade 2 spleen injury, a systolic blood pressure of 80, and respiratory rate of 12 who was 65 years old and has a GCS of 12 has a POS of 0.785. If you drop the GCS to 3, the POS changes to 0.273. The number of expected survivors in a population of trauma patients (for instance, a year's worth of patients at a trauma center) is done by adding the POS of all patients generating an *expected* number of survivors. This can then be compared to the actual number of survivors (actual survivors-expected survivors). The difference if negative indicated less patients survived than expected, a positive number indicated more survivors than predicted. A w score [5] can also be calculated using TRISS with the following equation ((actual expected survivors)/number of patients in population/100). A positive w indicated the number of excess survivors per 100 patients treated and a negative the number of expected survivors who would die in your trauma center per 100 patients.

There are several problems with TRISS that we will not go into here. They include the fact that TRISS was developed over 30 years ago, and some of the variables used are not considered suitable to encompass all the factors that affect mortality in trauma patients (for instance, there is no weight allowed for the patient's comorbidities). Also there are rules for whether certain vital signs are allowed in the calculation, such that if an immediate blood pressure or respiratory rate is not collected and recorded on arrival in the ED, then the POS should not be calculated due to the risk of inaccuracy (patient may have already received resuscitation).

For these reasons, other systems were created. Probably the most widely used in the USA is the Trauma Quality Improvement Project (TQIP) created by the American College of Surgeons (https://www.facs.org/quality-programs/trauma/tqp/center-programs/tqip). This is a system that is updated quarterly that uses a very large database of trauma patients from trauma centers throughout the USA and

Canada. Special training is given to registrars who enter data in TQIP at the trauma centers, and there are extensive validation systems.

No benchmarking system is perfect and we recommend using at least two systems. For instance, we use TRISS since it can provide immediate data (TQIP only provides quarterly reports that are 4 months behind the actual data) and TQIP to compare ourselves to our peers.

There are other benchmarking systems available to trauma centers. Many academic centers are members of the Vizient consortium (www.vizientinc.com). This is a purchasing and data analysis corporation that uses a proprietary system for comparing hospital performance. There are also other companies that have created trauma benchmarking systems and states that have developed their own systems. Every trauma center should (or must if verified by ACS) use a benchmarking system with risk adjustment methods.

Using These Systems and Analyzing Reports

Firstly, no benchmarking system is perfect. Any sufficiently important metric (especially when money is involved) will be gamed. If you look at the performance over time for systems where there are consequences for poor performance, improvement may be attributed to improvements in care, but it would be naïve to think that is the only factor at work. As an example, when the University HealthSystem Consortium (now Vizient) started grading academic medical centers based on their mortality rates, vigorous efforts were made to examine relevant clinical issues such as misdiagnosis, failure to escalate, failure to rescue, and medical error. However, almost equal effort was put into finding ways to remove patients who died from the accounting by creating real and virtual hospice units. When a patient was heading toward death, hospitals began "transferring" these patients to hospice units. Thus the patient was discharged from the treating hospital alive and not dead since they needed to be readmitted to the hospice unit. In some hospitals, "virtual" hospice units were created wherein the patient was discharged from the primary hospital and readmitted to hospice while staying in the same bed. This is just one example among many of how performance can be enhanced without improving clinical care.

But these systems provide many benefits. What I wrote above should not dissuade you from using benchmarking but should make you aware that your score, especially in comparison to hospitals that are gaming the metric, should not be viewed as the final word on your performance. What is more important is to examine your own performance in these metrics over time. By doing that, you should be able to discern opportunity for improvement that you can act upon.

References

1. Boyd CR, Tolson MA, Copes WS. Evaluating trauma care: the TRISS method. J Trauma. 1987;27:370.
2. Champion HR, Sacco WJ, Carnazzo AJ, et al. Trauma Score. Crit Care Med. 1980;9:672.
3. Baker SP, O'Neill B, Haddon W, et al. The injury severity score: A method for describing patients with multiple injuries and evaluating emergency care. J Trauma. 1974;14:187.
4. Champion HR, Sacco WJ, Hunt TK. Trauma severity scoring to predict mortality. World J Surg. 1983;7(1):4–11.
5. Champion HR, Sacco WJ, Copes WS. Improvement in outcome from trauma center care. Arch Surg. 1992;127(3):333–8.

Chapter 16
Putting It Together: Carrying Out Focused Improvement

Case Studies

Undertriage

Undertriage is the common opportunity for improvement in many trauma centers. Due to variability in the capabilities of prehospital providers and referring centers, inaccurate information can be provided to the trauma center leading to an inaccurate classification of the incoming patient. For this reason, every center, even the most experienced and mature, has cases of undertriage. The key finding in the performance review process when examining undertriage is to determine whether it is an underlying serious problem in this process or just an episode of sloppy thinking and inaccurate information.

As a broad example, let's say that your Level II trauma center patient comes in and the patient's initial blood pressure was 120/80 and pulse of 90, but when examined by the emergency medicine physician on the ED, the patient was hypotensive, tachycardic and in deep shock. At this point, a trauma activation is initiated, but the trauma team is somewhat

© Springer Nature Switzerland AG 2020
J. S. Young, *Trauma Centers*,
https://doi.org/10.1007/978-3-030-34607-2_16

behind the curve, and they are arriving 5–10 minutes after the patient has already been in the emergency department. In this case, usually, there are delays in blood administration and the resuscitation tends to be disjointed and inefficient. In severe cases, if the condition of the patient is not rapidly recognized, there can be an unexpected mortality.

When examining a case like this, go back to the source information. What was the original prehospital report or the report from the referring hospital? Was the change in condition evident prior to arrival at the trauma center? Was the change in condition properly communicated to the trauma center and was this information related to the people who can activate the trauma team? It is important that the PI program investigates this as soon as possible to the event so that frangible information is not lost. For the sake of illustration, in this case, it was found that the prehospital medic unit called in when they were 5 minutes from the trauma center with evidence of a patient who was now in hypotensive shock. It is unclear who received this transmission even though you have documentation that the transmission occurred. It is also unclear if someone received this information and was it relayed to the appropriate people. Through further investigation you find that the trauma center does not have someone stationed at the prehospital radio in the emergency department, and it is common for people to answer the radio were just passing by. You find there is no standard process for answering the prehospital radio, and the people who do answer are not properly trained in the trauma activation criteria and the process for activating trauma team. Your corrective action is to work with the emergency department to develop standard work for monitoring the prehospital radio system and for streamlining the process for activating the alert. You then audit this process by episodes of undertriage for the next 6 months to ensure that the OFIs do not recur.

This is a rather simple straightforward and easy to address opportunity for improvement from triage, but there are far more complicated ones. For example, some trauma centers do not have the physician/surgeon resources to respond appro-

priately to patients meeting the highest level activation criteria created by the American College of Surgeons. In examining
undertriage at these centers, you will encounter evidence that
the emergency medicine physicians downplay the physiologic
derangement of patients from prehospital and referring hospital reports in order not to unduly overwork their surgeons
who are taking trauma call. This is especially evident in centers where they are using surgeons who may practice at multiple hospitals and surgeons who are not in-house at night. In
those instances, the emergency medicine physicians often are
pressured to only activate the trauma team when there is no
question that the criteria have been met. For those cases
where the letter of the law of the criteria may be met, but it is
a judgment call, they will often err on the side of not activating the team. It would be important that the PI program at
these centers examine whether this process is hurting patients.
If it is hurting patients, then they must stop it. As a site visitor,
you will often see evidence of this undertriage and there is
clear documentation that the patient met activation criteria.
You discern from the PI process that the emergency medicine
physician, or emergency department nurse was making
excuses as to why they did not activate the team such as "you
can never trust that medic unit they provide information,"
"the referring hospital always exaggerates what's wrong with
patients in order to get them transferred quickly," etc. You
would expect the trauma program staff to address these sorts
of issues aggressively since they can seriously alter the outcome of injured patients.

Procedural/Operating Room Unavailability

Every trauma center has to walk the fine line between excessive resource utilization and the ability to respond to critically injured patients in a timely fashion. The American
College of Surgeons requires an operating room team in-
house at all times with another team that responds to the
hospital if the on-call team becomes encumbered.

Interventional radiology response needs to occur within 30 minutes notification. There will be instances when the system is overwhelmed, but the site visit team will be looking for delays in care during normal operations.

As an example, a patient arrives with a stab wound to the abdomen and a systolic blood pressure of 90 mm hg. There is a highest-level trauma activation, and the team meets them in the ED. They arrive at 815 AM on a Tuesday when all elective OR cases have begun. When the operating room is contacted to immediately bring patient up, they state no room is available, all elective cases have begun, and add-on cases were placed in the discretionary rooms. The estimate wait is 1 hour. The patient requires blood products during the delay and suffers an acute kidney injury postoperatively.

In this case, this is an unacceptable delay. If three stab wound patients arrived at the same time and there was a 1-hour delay, then perhaps, after PI review, this would be deemed unavoidable, but a 1-hour delay for a stab wound with questionable stability is unacceptable. The PI program should begin with the basics: was a highest level activation called? Did the OR receive it? What did they do when they received it? Was the standard work for room availability (keeping a discretionary or a "flex" room available at all times) not done?

Assuming the communication was solid, but that the OR just did not follow the standard work for staggering starts to insure there is always a room available, the PI process should document that the standard work was carried out in the usual fashion. At this point, they would focus on the operating room and their process of insuring a room is always available for critical trauma patients. Could a room have been available faster? Was the severity of the patient's condition properly communicated? The PI process should individually interview the involved anesthesiologists or operating room staff, or a root cause analysis-type meeting could be done with all the relevant frontline personnel in the room at the same time.

In investigations of this type it should be stressed that no one is looking to blame anyone, that the purpose of this process is to identify defects in the process. By encouraging honesty and transparency the PI program can have a realistic appraisal of their systems and make them better. Let's assume that in this case, there was just a confluence of circumstances that led to a room not being available at 8:15 in the morning on a weekday. This situation is in some ways the essence of performance improvement. The program should work with the operating room to understand their limitations in having a room available and make an assessment of whether the situation represented such a rare event that it should simply be monitored and that the standard work was functioning optimally. This can be assessed by looking at the time from patient arrival to OR arrival for a variety of critical patients during high-level activations. If it is determined that there is actually a problem with the process, the Plan-Do-Study-Act Method for correcting the defect should be used. As an example, the OR and the trauma program staff can work together to look at how standard work for staggering starts can improve the process. Also they should review the literature to see what best practice for this process entails. In general a staggered start process is all that is needed (a room does not need to be held at all times).

Neurosurgical Absence

There is a shortage of neurosurgeons nationwide, and the trauma center requirements for neurosurgical consultation and treatment are fairly strict. Very few hospitals have more neurosurgeons than they need, and often many communities require neurosurgeons to work at more than one hospital. This can lead to problems when immediate neurosurgical consultation is needed.

As a case example, an 89-year-old patient on blood thinners arrives at a Level II trauma center after a ground-level fall. The patient is seen at an outside hospital and they exhibit altered mental status and a subdural hematoma with a width of 1 cm and 1 mm of midline shift is found on imaging of the head. The patient is awake but disoriented and moves all extremities. This is classified as a second-level activation, and the trauma team is present on arrival. When the call from the transfer hospital arrived, the trauma surgeon asked that neurosurgery be informed and was told that the neurosurgeon was in the operating room. When the patient arrives, the mental status is far worse than advertised, and the patient requires immediate intubation. The patient is then taken to the CT scanner where it is found that the subdural hematoma has doubled in size and the midline shift is far worse. Neurosurgery is called immediately but is still in the operating room. When the trauma surgeon attempts to contact the backup neurosurgeon on the schedule, they cannot be reached. The neurosurgeon is contacted in the operating room is asked what we should do? He states that the patient now needs to go to another hospital. The patient undergoes medical management of suspect intracranial hypertension and is transferred to Level I trauma center 30 miles away. The patient has a poor neurologic outcome and dies.

This is a critical case for performance improvement review, and site reviewers that will examine the PI programs response very carefully. Needless to say the trauma program team should extend a great deal of effort into examining and correcting the defects in this case.

As always the PI process should begin with a review of the facts. These are examples:

- The information received from the referring hospital
- The information that was presented to the neurosurgeon prior to arrival
- An interview with the OR staff to ensure that this information was properly given to the nurse in the room with the neurosurgeon
- A discussion with the neurosurgeon as to whether they attempted to contact backup when they knew they might be encumbered when the patient arrived

- An examination of previous cases where neurosurgical response may have been delayed

The corrective action plan would depend on the findings, but the process should be thoroughly documented. The program should be able to answer the question "if the same situation happened again today, would we know that the patient would get more expeditious care? And how would we know that?" It would be expected that the program should audit neurosurgical response for a period of time to ensure whatever corrective actions were put in place have been effective.

This case might also open up some serious issues for a trauma center regarding neurosurgical commitment. Seeing a case like this, the site reviewers would focus on the center's neurosurgical commitment and would probably directly interview the neurosurgery liaison to see how much they supported the mission of the trauma center. This is why it is incredibly important for the trauma program to make a tremendous effort in examining this case and demonstrating that they understand it's importance and will expend significant effort to ensure it does not happen again. The PI process in this case should all be thoroughly documented in the records. As well as the records from the PI meetings.

Floor Mortality from Sedation

Morbidity from oversedation is a common adverse event in hospitals. Often inexperienced providers are responsible for sedation orders in the middle of the night, and these are often done over the phone. Occasionally, nursing staff is frustrated by an agitated patient when they have several other patients to take care of. They can push for sedatives that may cause respiratory depression, and the inexperienced physician may order them. In addition covering for patients you're not familiar with, especially those with pre-existing respiratory dysfunction can lead to poor decision making.

In this case, we are in a Level I trauma center at 2 o'clock in the morning and in the intermediate care unit when a 75-year-old patient with bilateral rib fractures and an acetabular fracture suddenly becomes agitated. The nurse contacts the resident on call and informs them of the situation. The resident asks for the patient's oxygen saturations and glucose and whether he/she received any meds within the last hour. The patient's saturations are 95%, glucose is 100, and he/she had not received any sedation the past hour. The resident orders 2 mg of Versed IV. The nurse calls back 30 minutes later and says that the patient now has pulled out there IV and is trying to get out of bed. The resident orders 4 mg Versed IV and due to the patient's injuries orders 100 μg of fentanyl. Twenty minutes later, a rapid response team calls initiated for the patient's room. The resident arrives to find the patient being bagged by the nurse, with vomit on their chin and chest and oxygen saturations of 70%. The patient is subsequently intubated by anesthesia and transferred to the surgical intensive care unit where 5 days later he/she died due to sepsis.

Part IV
The Site Visit Process

Chapter 17
The Basics of State and ACS Site Visits

State Versus ACS Designation

Almost every state has a trauma center verification and designation process. In some states, the process is immature and does not hold centers to a high standard, and others rival or exceed the standards set by the American College of Surgeons Committee on Trauma (COT).

An inspection process is the key element in a statewide trauma system. Without receiving hospitals that are known to provide state-of-the-art resuscitation and injury treatment, care of the injured in that area is determined by luck and whoever might be on call that night. The designation process allows prehospital and other facilities to know the capabilities of the accepting center and that those capabilities are available 24/7/365. The COT developed the verification review system over 25 years ago and has completed thousands of inspections across the USA and in a few foreign countries. The standard of the COT, written in the document "Optimal Resources for the Care of the Injured Patient" (https://www.facs.org/quality-programs/trauma/tqp/center-programs/vrc/resources) [1], is consistently

© Springer Nature Switzerland AG 2020   191
J. S. Young, *Trauma Centers*,
https://doi.org/10.1007/978-3-030-34607-2_17

reviewed and updated. I have been a member of the committee responsible for this process for almost 20 years and have completed over 160 ACS site visits, with the vast majority in Level I and II centers. In over 90% of these reviews, I functioned as the senior reviewer who is responsible for the conduct of the visit and for the accuracy and fairness of the report.

In my opinion, with this large amount of experience, ACS-verified centers provide more consistent care than most state-verified centers (except perhaps for the excellent systems in Pennsylvania run by the Pennsylvania Trauma Systems Foundation and the state of Maryland). Level I centers tend to be very consistent, primarily with differences in the PI process. Level II centers tend to have the highest amount of variability.

Any center that wishes to demonstrate they meet an accepted national standard of excellence for care of the injured patient should make the necessary investment to be verified by the ACS. This is no way means that centers only verified by their states are providing a lower level of care, but ACS verification is a consistent standard of personal, administrative, and financial commitment to trauma care. In addition, the ACS process requires a benchmarking system which as I have written is critical to evaluating the level of care provided.

Deciding Whether You Are Prepared for an ACS Site Visit

A center should be far along the path of functioning as a trauma center before undergoing an ACS COT site visit. This often requires 3–5 years of planning, administrative commitment, recruitment, and education of staff. The basic structure of a verifiable trauma center is outlined in the previous parts of this book and will not be repeated.

The Consultative Visit

Centers that are unsure of their capabilities can request a consultative visit from the ACS. Few states provide this service. The ACS will assign two senior trauma surgeons and an experienced trauma program manager, all from verified centers, to conduct the visit. The process for the consultative visit is identical to a verification visit (chart review, dinner, tour, interviews, and exit interview), but the team will endeavor to be extremely concrete about adherence to criteria. If the team does not pick up something that a follow-up verification team cites as a deficiency, then the consultative team has failed in its purpose. This is why few centers complete consultative visits with less than 6–8 deficiencies (and I have done consultative visits with over 60 deficiencies). This does not mean we are more lenient during the verification visit. This means that if there is any possibility whatsoever that a process will be given a deficiency during a verification visit, we will make it a deficiency in the consultative visit.

Some state-verified centers (including my own) opted to undergo a verification visit without a consultation first. Realistically, this should only be done if a member of the center has extensive experience with the ACS process (for instance, working in a previously ACS-verified center). The reasons are that though the ACS provides excellent guidance for centers being visited, there are many subtle issues (such as how to set up charts, prepare your liaisons for the visit, etc.) that cannot be fully understood if no one in leadership has been through or observed an ACS visit.

Contacting the ACS Office

The capabilities of the ACS to do visits have increased tremendously over the past two decades through the training of additional reviewers. While it was not unusual to wait

18 months to have a visit in the past, visits can now be scheduled in a shorter time frame in most cases. But it is important to contact the ACS office as early as possible to gain access to the pre-review questionnaire (PRQ) and begin to insure that your PI program meets ACS standards. Specific instructions and necessary materials are found on this website (https://www.facs.org/quality-programs/trauma/tqp/center-programs/vrc) [2].

Filling Out the Pre-review Questionnaire (PRQ)

Your first and most important task is to fill out the PRQ. This is the document your reviewers will examine prior to the visit and will often determine what areas they will take a strong interest in. Inconsistencies, grammatical errors, incoherent entries, and blank sections will always raise suspicions about the diligence and level of involvement of senior staff.

You will most likely need to split up the PRQ and have different sections filled out by different personnel; however, there should be one person responsible for editing and signing off on the document. Do not confabulate or attempt to hide issues in the PRQ. The senior reviewer will not only be a TMD or associate TMD at an ACS-verified center, but the junior reviewer is often very experienced as well. Trauma directors are well aware of trouble spots and will often go to those sections of the PRQ that reveal the most about the program (usually section V, trauma service, and section XVI, performance improvement and patient safety). If the visitors encounter untruths, they will immediately be suspicious that many areas of the document are dubious and will drill down and ask for confirmatory paperwork for everything in the document, rather than spot-checking. I have been in several visits where the program attempted to cover up deficiencies, and it did not work out well. Many times, these issues involve problems that the program has tried to solve (backup neurosurgery and orthopedic call, for instance) and have been unsuccessful due to lack of support from the hospital and other specialties. The inability to solve these problems demonstrates a lack of commitment on the part of the hospital and clinical staff and thus would warrant a critical deficiency.

Have each section reviewed by two people with extensive knowledge of the program. Insure that the numbers in all tables add up correctly (or you will be asked to redo them and to explain discrepancies) and that any areas where you may be in danger of receiving a deficiency are thoroughly outlined. Often a reviewer will view an issue differently if the program demonstrates honesty and commitment throughout. A very useful effect of an ACS visit is that an outside group citing a deficiency is often a very effective means to compel the hospital to provide the necessary support.

Do not be overly verbose. Unfortunately, the document prints in such a way that overly long answers are difficult to follow. I recommend the use of bullet points to emphasize critical parts of a section. It makes the section easier to read and highlights important information, rather than having it buried in prose. Edit for grammatical issues and spelling errors. While these errors are not fatal, their presence demonstrates a sloppy effort in creating the document.

References

1. Committee on Trauma, American College of Surgeons. Resource for optimal care of the injured patient. 2014. https://www.facs.org/-/media/files/quality-programs/trauma/vrc-resources/resources-for-optimal-care.ashx?la=en
2. Committee on Trauma, American College of Surgeons. Verification, Review, and Consultation (VRC) Program. 2019. https://www.facs.org/quality-programs/trauma/tqp/center-programs/vrc. Accessed 25 Sept 2019.

Chapter 18
Preparing for the Visit

First, I want to stress that nothing I write here should override information coming from the ACS verification office. The ACS office in Chicago and the reviewers at your visit are the final authority on issues regarding the satisfaction of criteria. What I am providing is advice to help you through the process. These are my opinions and experiences and in no way represent official opinions of the ACS COT Verification Review Committee.

You should begin your preparation for the site visit at least 12 months before the scheduled date. If you are already verified, then you should know when your site visit year is and should contact the office 12–14 months ahead of your expiration date to set up your visit. At this point, you will determine what 12 months constitute your "site visit year." This 12-month period cannot be more than 16 months from your site visit date and obviously cannot be less than 12 months from that date. You should work with your registrar to determine how caught up your registry is and also look at your MDPI meeting attendance. If someone is at 30% attendance (the requirement being 50%), you need to

© Springer Nature Switzerland AG 2020
J. S. Young, *Trauma Centers*,
https://doi.org/10.1007/978-3-030-34607-2_18

try to give that person enough time to make up the missed sessions. Other strategies are to add a December meeting if there will be good turnout and to remove a meeting if you know there will be bad turnout for a certain month as this will hurt your attendance percentage.

You should have read through the latest version of the optimal resources document (https://www.facs.org/quality-programs/trauma/tqp/center-programs/vrc/resources) [1] and any other bulletins that were sent out by the ACS regarding criteria. There are also regular webinars put on by the verification office that can provide important information.

At this point (10–12 months prior to the scheduled visit), I would recommend that you take another thorough look at your major PI issues and determine how many are still open (have not achieved loop closure) and whether you have properly documented loop closure in those that you believe are complete. For those deaths and major PI cases going forward from the start of your site visit year, we recommend that you should begin to put these charts together in the format required for the visit. Here is a recommended structure for charts you will provide to the site visit team.

Use a manila (or similar) folder that has a locking clasp on the inside of both sides of the folder. On the left side (as you are facing the folder) place:

- Registry demographic sheet (be certain that the patient's ISS is on every chart in an easy to find location or place the name, age, category, and ISS on the chart label)
- PI evaluation form that clearly documents the path the case took through the process
- Emails, letters, and other documentation of the loop closure process including M&M meeting presentations, MDPI meeting minutes, hospital quality program documentation (if possible), etc.

Finally, a perfect chart will have a page with the patient information, the opportunity for improvement, the corrective action, and the documentation of loop closure.

On the right side:

- Prehospital records
- Emergency department flowsheet

  – Insure that time of arrival, time alert was called, alert this was a highest level activation, and documentation of trauma surgeon arrival time are highlighted

- Trauma service (or admitting service) history and physical
- Operative notes from first 24 hours
- Discharge summary
- Autopsy if available

The key to chart preparation is to tell a story to the reviewers. I have done visits where centers just printed 1000 pages of chart with no dividers or sections and no PI records so that we had to ask for them on every case. This does not make a good impression on the reviewers and simply indicates a lack of preparation and forethought about what the entire chart review is about.

The optimal situation is when the reviewers primarily use your own PI records to do their chart review, but bear in mind this will usually only be done in a mature center that has been through several visits. In that situation, they are trusting you to properly abstract and analyze the case. All reviewers will spot-check items in the record (time to OR, time to attending arrival, etc.), but the less that the reviewers go through every page of the record, the lower the chance they will find something that you didn't. Reviewers will look at every page when they have seen through the first few charts, or through the previous report, that the PI program has problems with issue identification. It is imperative that the way you set up the chart for review takes the reviewer from prehospital all the way through discharge and PI closure in a logical, easy to follow narrative.

In our own center, the TMD and associate TMD review every chart that we put in front of the reviewers to insure that each chart tells the story clearly. If we find problems, we correct them prior to the date of the visit. This is why it is beneficial to start putting together the charts well ahead of the visit so that you are not left with 100 charts to review for accuracy and flow 1 week before the visit. In our site visit year, we built charts from deaths and closed PI cases in a rolling fashion, and the leadership reviewed the completed charts every quarter. It is astounding to me that a TPM and/or TMD would not go through every page that is given to site reviewers prior to their visit.

Chart Review

There are ways for the chart review to go well and for it to go very poorly. The environment of the chart reviews can set you up for success or less than success.

First, the room where the charts are located for review should be large and seat at least ten people comfortably. Boardrooms and conference rooms are the most commonly used. Do not set up the chart reviews in an office (at some-one's desk as I once experienced), do not put the charts in a room separate from where the reviewers will sit, and do not set up in a room too small for the reviewers, charts, and trauma program staff. Provide lunch for the reviewers and the space to eat. If the reviewers are arriving in the morning, you should provide a simple breakfast. Provide soft drinks, water, coffee, and ice and locate the room within reasonable distance from a bathroom. You must also provide Internet access either through a guest network or a login to the secure network (with a temporary password if necessary). The form we fill out for the report is online and cannot be entered without Internet access. Provide the reviewers with login information immediately on arrival. Make certain the temperature in the room is comfortable if at all possible.

The charts should be neatly organized into boxes for each category (or several categories can be combined into one box if charts are small). Make sure each chart has a label on it with name, age, ISS, and category. It is also very helpful to place a sticker on the charts where there was PI program review. Remember that all deaths must have PI program review and documentation. If you have a com-pletely electronic medical record, you must at least print out the sections I detailed above and all PI records related to that case. Though some reviewers will not use them, you should have a computer set up with medical record access and staff at each computer to assist the reviewer.

Some things you should never do:

- Provide no printed out material such that the review must abstract everything from the computer.
- Not have EMR access in chart review room.
- Place printouts in charts without subdivision and labeling.
- Tell the reviewers "if you need the PI, we can get it." They will always need the PI, and they do not want to wait 10 minutes for you to find it on every chart. This demonstrates an immature program that has not prepared adequately.
- When the reviewers ask about a complex case, say "oh yeah, Jimmie, he was …" and then go off on a 5-minute monologue about the case. Provide the documentation to the reviewer and allow them to ask specific questions.
- Do not look over the reviewer's shoulder and read what they are writing or listen when reviewers are discussing issues unless they are including you in the conversation.
- Do not try to hide information from the reviewers and be completely honest about your mistakes. Every program misses an opportunity for improvement so if the reviewers find such a case, simply say you missed it, thanks for identifying the problem, and we will look into why it was missed and review the case. Do not say the documentation exists but you couldn't find it because if you do, the reviewers will tell you to find it to make sure you are being truthful. If this is a huge oversight (such as an unanticipated death with serious issues), then you may suffer some consequences regarding the evaluation of the PI program. But that is better than fabricating an excuse.

You need to stay with the reviewers for the first 30–60 minutes to insure they know their way around the charts and computerized records. Occasionally, 1–2 staff should stay with reviewers at all times (usually the trauma registrar, TPM/PI coordinator, and/or TMD), but do not use the chart review room as a meeting place for the entire staff. Do not have the staff sit around and talk loudly, answer their phones, check email, etc. while the reviewers are doing their work. This is incredibly distracting. If you do this, do not be surprised if the reviewers put earbuds in to block out the noise. Insure that the cell phone number of the TMD and TPM is easily visible to the team and that those people will come immediately if summoned.

A question often arises whether the TMD and TPM should stay with team at all times. My advice is that they should always be immediately available and should stay until told they can leave. Do not schedule operating room cases on the days of the visit. The team asks for about 8 hours of your time every 3 years. If you can't provide that without interruption, then your commitment to the program will be questioned. It looks extremely poor for the TMD to be unavailable during the visit and is always noticed.

Dinner

The site visit dinner is a chance for the trauma program to shine in front of the executive leadership of the hospital. Below is a briefing sheet that I provide to all liaisons and other trauma center personnel attending the dinner and who are involved in the tour the following day:

- Never argue with the reviewers please. If they identify something we did not anticipate, or we do not have a plan to improve an issue, just tell them we will make improvement in that area a priority.
- Please look over your area of responsibility; contact me for any questions or clarifications. Many of these questions will be asked at the dinner and the tour, please don't say we already answered that.
- Show up on time (late people are noticed by reviewers). Absent people are even more noticed and can turn a weakness into a deficiency if they see lack of engagement.
- If they have concerns about a part of the program (which we will have a hint from the chart review the afternoon of the dinner), it is absolutely essential that the person representing that part of the program be at the dinner or tour, on time, and engaged.

- We will eat during the questioning at the dinner, and the expectation is the dinner should take 90 minutes to 2 hours.
- *Conduct of the Dinner and Tour*

  - The reviewers run the show, no presentations or video or anything from us.
  - At dinner, they will first go around the table and ask everyone to introduce themselves.
  - They will verify the application document (PRQ); therefore, they will ask questions from each section. Below are the usual questions from each section and who usually answers. If there are questions specific to the tour, I have included them:

    - Section I – Purpose of visit and review of previous visit

      - This involves findings from previous visits; below are the weaknesses and recommendations from the last visit.
      - If these responses involve your area and you have any questions, please contact us this week.

    - Section II – Hospital information

      - We are the only Level 1 application I have ever seen where there are no other trauma centers of any level within 50 miles. They will inquire about this and how we coordinate care in this very large region.

        - Associate TMD and TPM should answer and describe our regional outreach efforts, our feedback to referring hospitals, our work with referring hospitals, and our cooperation at the state level with the other Level 1s in the state.

    - Section III – Prehospital

      - They will comment on Drs. A and B being involved as operational medical directors, which is very unusual as trauma surgeons. This will likely be cited as a strength.

    – They may ask about our aeromedical coverage
      and prehospital protocol development. Dr. X
      should handle these questions. We should also
      stress our MEDCOM program since this is a very
      unique and strength of our program.

- Section IV – Trauma service

    – This is a very large section and will take time.
      TMD and associate TMD should answer the
      majority of the questions.
    – They will ask us how the trauma service
      functions.
    – We will stress that trauma critical care is a sepa-
      rate ICU service which will likely be cited as a
      strength.
    – What is our NP coverage and our resident
      coverage?
    – They will ask about the nighttime ICU program
      and whether the in-house trauma attending could
      potentially be unavailable if called to be with a
      non-trauma patient.
    – They will ask D about her role.
    – Explain why the gamma alert was initiated and
      what value you think it provides? (Dr. B can
      answer.)
    – What are the requirements for an attending see-
      ing a beta and gamma alert? (Drs. A and B can
      answer.)
    – They will ask about how we evaluate nonsurgical
      admissions. Trauma registrar should start with
      how these patients are identified, PI coordinator
      should describe the process of analysis, and then
      the associate TMD should describe his role and
      how outliers are addressed.

- Most places have a diversion system; we will indicate we do not. Any diversion of major trauma from an ED or the scene is an error and not part of our policies; we examine every event and try to eliminate this from happening.
- Neurosurgery – they will ask Dr. N about how involved the NS attendings are in neurotrauma, how they insure consistent care, etc. They will also bring up issues with neurotrauma care found in chart review, if any are found.
- Orthopedics – Dr. O will need to describe how urgent cases are handled and what the involvement of the non-trauma ortho faculty is and also what patients are cared for by the ortho trauma attendings and which are not.

- Section V (most of these questions will be asked on the tour as well. Special tour considerations are included)

  - ED dinner

    - They will ask Drs. X and T about the relationship between the ED and trauma. It should be stressed that the EM residents spend several months on the trauma service during their residency.
    - They will ask why the ED attending needs to be in the loop when aeromedical, EMS, and other EDs call in patients who meet alpha and beta trauma alert criteria.
    - Tour

      - They will start with where the patient enters the system (helipad and ambulance parking area).
      - They will ask to see the decontamination room (make certain it is clean).
      - They will ask how we would conduct a mass decontamination event.

- They will then go to the trauma bay. The size of our bays will likely be cited as a weakness (we have construction plans as our response).
- They will go to the trauma bays

  - They will want to see inside our carts.
  - What training do the ED nurses and techs go through before they are allowed to be at the bedside of an alpha alert?
  - What is in the blood refrigerator?
  - Who goes with the trauma patient to CT?

- Radiology

  - They will ask Dr. R what our error rate is by ACR standards.
  - When are attendings in house reading films?
  - What is the process when the attending is not in house?
  - Are there any films the attending is required to read at night?
  - What is your IR response time from call to stick?
  - Tour

    - What CT is used for acute trauma?
    - How many slices?
    - Is it dedicated to the ED?
    - CT and MRI tech coverage at night?
    - They will likely cite the distance from our trauma bays to CT as a weakness (construction is corrective action).

- Operating room

  - What teams are here at 2 AM?
  - What is the anesthesiology coverage at 2 AM?
  - How do you arrange for a room for alpha alerts that need to come directly to the OR? (Dr. Anesthesia should answer this.)
  - Tour

    - If a gunshot wound to the abdomen with a BP of 60 was dropped off by personal vehicle at the ED at 8 AM on a Monday morning, what would you do? Show me how you would make a room for that patient at this moment.

- PACU (dinner and tour same questions)

  - Is there a PACU nurse 24/7?
  - Does the PACU serve as an ICU overflow? This means an established ICU patient being transfered from ICU to PACU due to bed needs. It does not usually mean a trauma patient coming out of the OR waiting for an ICU bed.

- ICU (dinner and tour same questions)

  - The trauma faculty should answer
  - What is the ICU resident and NP coverage for trauma ICU patients?
  - Who responds in the middle of the night?
  - How does the ICU PI process work?
  - ICU nursing certification is low and turnover rate is high. They will likely cite both of these as weaknesses. They will want to know what are our plans to improve these weaknesses.

- Blood bank

  - Describe your massive transfusion protocol.
  - We will describe fast blood and other improvements that have been made.
  - How do you know it is working and how do you make improvements?

    - TPM or associate TMD should answer.

  - Tour

    - How many units of O negative do you have in the blood bank at this moment?
    - Who is the regional blood bank?

- Section VI – Specialty services

  - Pediatric trauma

    - Pediatric surgery representative will answer.

- Describe the pediatric trauma system at UVa. Who responds to pediatric alpha alerts at midnight? How is care turned over?
- For a 12-year-old major trauma patient, who takes care of that patient in the PICU and how does communication work?

  - Geriatric trauma

    - We will describe gamma alert system.

  - Rehabilitation

    - How does the relationship with our rehabilitation hospital function?
    - What is the involvement of PM&R with trauma patients?

      - When do they see severe head injuries?
      - How do they coordinate with SW and PT/OT?

  - Spine

    - How is spine surgery coverage arranged?

  - Organ procurement

    - Relationship with OPO?
    - May be cited as strength

- Section VII – Performance improvement

  - They will not often go into extensive discussions about PI at the dinner, but they might.
  - Explain your PI process from issue identification to closure.
  - What are your most common loop-closure methods?
  - Explain how you formulate your IEP.
  - Give two examples of PI processes in the past year you are proud of.
  - What are your greatest gaps in performance?

- Section VIII – Education/outreach

  - Injury prevention coordinator

    - Tell us about a few of the injury prevention activities you are most proud of.

  - They will be very interested in Stop The Bleed courses
  - ATLS courses?
  - Paramedic and EMS education?

- Section IX – Research

  - Will likely be cited as a strength
  - Usually not discussed extensively at dinner

This covers the questions you can expect and that you should have more than just the TMD answering questions. It is important that attendees answer questions about their area.

Ask attendees to be 15 minutes early, since it does not look good for people to walk in late. Let me stress again, we are asking for 2 hours of people's time once every 3 years. Attendees need to realize how poor it looks when people are late or don't attend. The program should send out the night of the dinner 6 months ahead of time. A family vacation that was planned long before or a family emergency is a decent excuse as long as there is a proxy to fill in.

Your chief executive officer (CEO) should attend or the second in command. The CEO do not need to stay for the entire dinner (though it shows commitment to the trauma center if they do), but they should at the least come in and introduce themselves to the visitors. One thing that I've have seen happen that looks terrible is when the CEO comes in the middle of the dinner, interrupts the entire process, and then introduces themselves to the team and walks out. Do not do that.

Regarding the size and layout of the dinner, I have several pieces of advice. Be realistic about the number of attendees. If >25 people attend, then the size of the room becomes unwieldy. There should be the key members of the trauma program and surgeons and liaisons, executive leadership, blood bank, and rehabilitation at the least. In a combined adult and pediatric visit, it is possible to go over 30 people. For a layout, a square or rectangle with the reviewers in the middle of one side with the TMD and TPM on that side is optimal. Do not place people at multiple circular tables where the group will have their back to the reviewers. You can make a semicircle with the reviewers at a separate table, but this is somewhat unusual. Insure the reviewers have the equivalent of two spaces. We need to spread out our computers and materials, and doing this and dealing with dinner plates are difficult. Insure that the dinner can begin service at the start time of the dinner to minimize disruption in the middle of the dinner. Buffets work well since everyone can get up and get all their food, but you will need a 10-minute delay at that point when people fill their plates, which is tolerable. Also a buffet allows people to leave as soon as the reviewers are finished, rather than wait for a course or dessert. But plate service works as long as the staff have room to deliver the food and are not noisy or disruptive.

Tour

The tour is probably the least important part of the site visit. It's a process where you probably can't impress tremendously (since we've seen a lot of trauma centers), but the tour can cause problems. As in my briefing for the dinner and tour above, make certain the personnel who know the answers are available for the 30–45-minute time span where the reviewers will reach that unit. It reflects poorly on program when no one is available to answer questions when the reviewers arrive on a unit. I have experienced uncomfortable situations when the manager of the area was unavailable and the TPM grabbed whoever was nearby to answer questions and this person had no idea what was going on.

You should discuss with each person answering questions any problems that the reviewers may find (construction and closed room/ORs, etc.), and they should have at hand the corrective actions to physical plant issues. In many hospitals, the ED is far from CT and the OR and the ICU. Some reviewers will cite this as a weakness, but you are not likely to rebuild your hospital based on our comments. A good response is that "we know this is a problem and we are working with hospital leadership to address it." New EDs tend to address many of these problems, but you need to make do with what you have.

Exit Interview

If the reviewers are doing their job correctly, there should be no surprises in the exit interview. I trained all the reviewers who have done site visits with me that they should choose a time usually 45–60 minutes prior to the exit interview to meet with the TPM and TMD and go over their findings. It is not necessary in this meeting to go over all the strengths of the program, but it is necessary to go over deficiencies and weaknesses. It is important that the program leadership understand the problems that were identified because understanding is the first step in correction. You also do not want a contentious situation at the exit interview since that does not serve any good purpose.

I will usually go over each individual weakness and our reasoning. If possible I'd like to go back to the original documentation that led to a decision. If you are assigning weaknesses or deficiencies based on the chart review, it is important to be specific about what chart indicated the problem. A common event is that during this briefing, when specific findings are presented, the program leadership will often be able to find additional documentation that addresses the concerns. This does not happen all the time but it is important to be as specific as possible with the program leadership so that they can find answers to your questions if they were not in the materials that have already been provided.

There are instances where the program will simply not accept your findings. In these situations, it is important for the senior reviewer to take control and calmly, logically, and unemotionally explain to the program why you reached these conclusions and tell them that there is a process by which they can appeal your findings to the ACS. These are rare events if the site visit is conducted properly. This occurs in most situations when the program knew they were out of compliance and hoped that the site visit team would simply ignore the issue. The checks and balances built into the site review process, wherein the report is peer reviewed by the committee, make it virtually impossible for a site visit team to overlook something significant in the hopes that it will not be found. The peer reviewers often read the reports very carefully, as well as the cases, and any glaring issue will need to be addressed after the visit with the site visit team. There are instances where the peer reviewers bring up issues that the site reviewer disagrees with, and in those cases, majority of the time, the senior reviewer is felt to hold sway over the issue.

It is not necessary to have a huge crowd at the exit interview. In fact I think that unless you are certain that your report is going to be glowing, I would only have the program leadership, administrative leadership, and possibly executive suite representation at the exit interview. I would also advise the program leadership that if there are negative parts of the report, they should inform the executive leadership of this before the exit interview because you also do not want them to be surprised at that moment.

Reference

1. Committee on Trauma, American College of Surgeons. Resources for optimal care of the injured patient 2014/resources repository. 2019.   https://www.facs.org/quality-programs/trauma/tqp/center-programs/vrc/resources. Accessed 25 Sept 2019.

Chapter 19
Dealing with the Site Visit Findings

Corrective Actions

The criteria that the ACS uses to determine suitability for trauma center verification are classified as type 1 and type 2. A single type 1 criteria deficiency prevents verification; a center needs >3 type 2 deficiencies to prevent verification (visit this webpage for more information https://www.facs.org/quality-programs/trauma/tqp/center-programs/vrc/outcomes) [1]. If three or less type 2 deficiencies are found, the center is given a 1-year certificate of verification, and the center must correct the deficiencies within 12 months. If they are corrected, a 3-year verification is granted starting from the date of the notification. If a type 1 or >3 type 2 deficiencies are found, a focused review is required in order to be granted a verification certificate.

Weaknesses are more variable and often left to the discretion of the site visit team. However, weaknesses that are far outside of the usual practice of the verification review committee are routinely removed through the peer review process. For instance, if a weakness is cited that appears purely to be the result of a single reviewer's preference, this will usually

© Springer Nature Switzerland AG 2020
J. S. Young, *Trauma Centers*,
https://doi.org/10.1007/978-3-030-34607-2_19

be removed. A great deal time is put into creating and validating the criteria that are used. In general, weaknesses should be addressed before the next visit. There is no number of weaknesses that prohibit verification. However, if a center has a tremendous number of weaknesses, this can be a red flag to the verification review committee that there are significant problems at the center, and it is possible that a weakness could be elevated to a deficiency in consultation with the site visit team. This is why at the beginning of the exit interview, an exit interview statement is read by the reviewers that describes the process after the review was concluded. Basically, it states that the findings that are talked about in the exit interview may not be the findings that end up in the final report and that deficiencies can be made into weaknesses and vice versa. Both things do occur but not frequently. In general the committee should trust the opinion of the site reviewers who are on the ground and usually will only overrule them when it is clear from their report that the deficiency or weakness should or should not be cited.

Some centers view weaknesses and type II criteria deficiencies as "suggestions." This is not true. All criteria deficiencies must be corrected by the next visit, and centers with more than three type II deficiencies must correct them within 12 months. All type I deficiencies must be corrected within 12 months as well. While the type II criteria may be less directly related to the critical aspects of care of the injured patient, they are still felt to be essential components of a trauma center. For instance, many Level II centers that are attempting to be verified as a Level I centers will receive type II deficiencies for inadequate research productivity. This can be a very high hurdle to get over since if they have more than three type 2s and this is one of them, it is difficult to generate three to four manuscripts in publication in a 12-month period. This is why it is so important for centers to do a rational assessment of their center before determining on what level trauma center they wish to become. The verification review committee is very concrete when it comes to meeting all of the quantitative criteria. Performance improvement can be more qualitative, but that is the reason why reviewers are experienced TPMs and TMDs whose own centers have undergone verification.

It is important to begin addressing deficiencies and weaknesses immediately after the visit. There are some deficiencies that simply require sending paperwork to the VRC office. This includes call schedules that were not available during the visit, other documentation of board certification, etc. After your visit, you should communicate with the main office as to what is required to satisfy criteria deficiencies that merely require verification of paperwork.

There are some non-paperwork type II deficiencies that can also be addressed without a focused visit, and this should be discussed with the main office after the visit. Type I deficiencies always require a focused visit by a site visit team. While it is preferable for the same team to do the focus visit if they did the initial visit, it is not absolutely mandatory. And if the center felt that one member of the initial visit team was evaluating them in an unfair manner, that should absolutely be brought to the attention of the verification program manager, and they will endeavor to identify another reviewer to come back for your focused review. However, remember that the reports are not only reviewed by the junior and senior reviewer, they are also reviewed by a subset of the verification review committee, the trauma verification program manager, and the chair and/or vice chair of the verification review committee. So it is difficult for a single reviewer to unfairly evaluate a center such that they would not be verified.

I recommend that if you received serious deficiencies, especially for PI, you should continue to have contact with your senior reviewer or the reviewer that evaluated your PI program. You should discuss with them specifically what deficiencies they found in your performance improvement process and what they would expect to demonstrate compliance, and they should be able to provide you with concrete examples of how to meet these expectations. If they are not easy to communicate with, do not hesitate to contact the committee through the program manager or the chair and vice chair.

Every senior reviewer should be willing to thoroughly explain why they gave a deficiency and help the program define what is necessary to correct the issue.

Reference

1. Committee on Trauma, American College of Surgeons. Site visit outcomes. 2019. https://www.facs.org/quality-programs/trauma/tqp/center-programs/vrc/outcomes. Accessed 25 Sept 2019.

Index

© Springer Nature Switzerland AG 2020
J. S. Young, *Trauma Centers*,
https://doi.org/10.1007/978-3-030-34607-2